DIVERSITY on the EXECUTIVE PATH

DIVERSITY on the
EXECUTIVE
PATH

Wisdom and Insights for Navigating to the Highest Levels of Healthcare Leadership

Diane L. Dixon

ACHE Management Series

Your board, staff, or clients may also benefit from this book's insight. For information on quantity discounts, contact the Health Administration Press Marketing Manager at (312) 424-9450.

This publication is intended to provide accurate and authoritative information in regard to the subject matter covered. It is sold, or otherwise provided, with the understanding that the publisher is not engaged in rendering professional services. If professional advice or other expert assistance is required, the services of a competent professional should be sought.

The statements and opinions contained in this book are strictly those of the author and do not represent the official positions of the American College of Healthcare Executives or the Foundation of the American College of Healthcare Executives.

24 23 22 21 20   5 4 3 2

Library of Congress Cataloging-in-Publication Data
Names: Dixon, Diane L., author.
Title: Diversity on the executive path : wisdom and insights for navigating to the highest levels of healthcare leadership / Diane L. Dixon.
Other titles: Management series (Ann Arbor, Mich.)
Description: Chicago, IL : Health Administration Press, [2020] | Series: HAP/ACHE management series | Includes bibliographical references and index. | Summary: "This book is about the lived experiences on the executive path of 12 racially and ethnically diverse hospital and health system CEOs. It is based on interviews. It seeks to learn from the collective wisdom of all the executives to provide a unique glimpse, from their perspectives, into what it takes to navigate the challenges and opportunities of the executive path to the C-suite"— Provided by publisher.
Identifiers: LCCN 2019029654 (print) | ISBN 9781640551206 (paperback ; alk. paper) | ISBN 9781640551213 (ebook) | ISBN 9781640551237 (epub) | ISBN 9781640551244 (mobi) | ISBN 9781640551220 (xml)
Subjects: MESH: Health Facility Administrators | Leadership | Cultural Diversity | Professionalism | Organizational Culture | Organizational Objectives | United States
Classification: LCC RA971 (print) | LCC RA971 (ebook) | NLM WX 155 | DDC 362.1068/4—dc23
LC record available at https://lccn.loc.gov/2019029654
LC ebook record available at https://lccn.loc.gov/2019029655

The paper used in this publication meets the minimum requirements of American National Standard for Information Sciences—Permanence of Paper for Printed Library Materials, ANSI Z39.48-1984. ∞ ™

Acquisitions editor: Jennette McClain; Manuscript editor: Deborah Ring; Project manager: Andrew Baumann; Cover designer: James Slate; Layout: Integra

Found an error or a typo? We want to know! Please e-mail it to hapbooks@ache.org, mentioning the book's title and putting "Book Error" in the subject line.

For photocopying and copyright information, please contact Copyright Clearance Center at www.copyright.com or at (978) 750-8400.

Health Administration Press
A division of the Foundation of the American
   College of Healthcare Executives
300 S. Riverside Plaza, Suite 1900
Chicago, IL 60606-6698
(312) 424-2800

To my mother and father—thank you for the sacrifices that made it possible for me to be who and where I am today.

Contents

Foreword

MOST PEOPLE FROM racial and ethnic minority groups grow up hearing exactly the same messages about how to be successful in America. "Work hard!" In fact, we learn to expect to work twice as hard as everyone else. "Treat others with respect"—even when you don't receive the same respect. And my personal favorite: "Act with integrity and be true to your word."

I believe strongly in these virtues. Yet, in my experience, more is required of racially and ethnically diverse professionals to reach and lead at the top level in an organization. Diane L. Dixon, EdD, has been curious for decades about the "more" to which I refer. In *Diversity on the Executive Path: Wisdom and Insights for Navigating to the Highest Levels of Healthcare Leadership,* she explores whether racial and ethnic minorities confront more challenges than their majority counterparts do in entering the C-suite. Her research is substantive and validates some truths known by those of us who have successfully worked through these barriers.

Is leadership diversity in healthcare as critical now? This is an important conversation to have—truthfully and without judgment. With a small number of racially and ethnically diverse professionals rising to all levels of leadership in all facets of the healthcare field, a prevailing thought seems to be that we've moved past the need to focus on advocating for the growth of diverse leadership in management. I disagree. According to the American Hospital Association's Institute for Diversity and Health Equity, only 9 percent of hospital CEOs are minorities. At best, this is a static number that does not reflect the racially and ethnically diverse talent in the field or the communities served by healthcare organizations across this country. At worst, it is a number less than what it was just a couple of years ago.

Throughout her book, Dr. Dixon underscores the fact that diverse leadership is vital to the success of healthcare organizations and that we must have this difficult discussion, hire diverse leaders, create a diverse pipeline, and focus on retention and succession. Diverse representation at all levels, and particularly in governance and the C-suite, guides diversity in decision-making, strengthens healthcare through innovation and enhanced quality, and improves the equity in that care. Further, diversity of thought yields the best strategies and the best solutions.

Fortunately, Dr. Dixon goes beyond identifying the value of leadership diversity and the challenges to attaining it. She shares characteristics and competencies needed to achieve and thrive in executive roles. Although I continue to take advantage of opportunities to share my journey with professionals and students seeking advice and mentorship, I can touch only a limited number of people. Through this book, Dr. Dixon has compiled a road map to success that allows anyone interested in an ambitious career path in healthcare to explore strategies—and, most importantly, to build the leadership acumen that goes beyond the traditional requirements. She helps us look at the skills required to navigate in a society laced with unconscious and conscious color and ethnic bias.

One of the prevailing themes examined in this book is relationships—building them to bridge the gap and nurturing them through mentorship. As the CEO of CommonSpirit Health, the nation's largest nonprofit health system, I appreciate the complexity of the journey to the C-suite for members of underrepresented minority groups, as well as what it takes to sustain a successful career as a healthcare executive. In my more than 40 years in healthcare, I learned long ago the power of establishing authentic relationships by finding common ground with those who are different from yourself.

I wish the world were different now, but it isn't. I wish we could move past focusing on the need for diversity, but we can't. That is why I am particularly appreciative to Dr. Dixon for advancing this important discussion. Her research validates findings and provides real options to parlay what may otherwise feel like a stagnant career into one with a trajectory to a top management position.

—Kevin E. Lofton, FACHE
CEO, CommonSpirit Health

Preface

THE INSPIRATION FOR this research and this book began more than 22 years ago, when I was working on my doctoral degree in the Executive Leadership in Human and Organizational Learning program at George Washington University. During that time, I became interested in studying top leaders because of my experiences working as director of human resource development for two hospitals that were then part of a small health system. In that role, I was responsible for management and leadership development for department heads and supervisors. To support that work, I created an internal consulting service to help those leaders manage the many changes that were occurring in the hospitals. I worked with the hospitals' top executives, including the CEOs, to ensure that their development programs and organizational change processes were aligned with their expectations and with the overall strategy of the hospitals and health system. That experience gave me the opportunity to see firsthand the impact that the CEOs and top executive teams had on the hospitals and health system.

As a result, I focused my doctoral studies on leadership. I had a keen interest in learning more about effective leadership and its benefits for hospitals and health systems. My dissertation focused on the relationship between chief executive leadership (transactional and transformational) and hospital effectiveness. While identifying the research participants for my dissertation, I realized that very few racially and ethnically diverse professionals were hospital and health system CEOs. The CEOs whom I interviewed for my dissertation research were not racially and ethnically diverse. This concerned me, and I began to wonder: How did the few racially and ethnically diverse professionals who achieved that level of leadership get there?

That question was not the focus of my dissertation, however, and I wanted to complete my degree. After doing that in 1997 and becoming an independent leadership and organization development consultant, I continued to be interested in the underrepresentation of racially and ethnically diverse professionals in healthcare C-suites.

This interest was heightened some years later when I began teaching a Healthcare Leadership and Communications course in the Master of Health Services Administration program at the University of Maryland School of Public Health. Since I began teaching this course, I have found limited literature on diverse healthcare leaders and leadership. The literature that exists is even more limited in its attention to how racially and ethnically diverse professionals who have achieved executive leadership positions have done so. I have diverse students who are interested in achieving leadership positions at some point in their careers. But scarce resources are available to help them understand the executive path and apply that learning to their own careers. This information is not included in the standard leadership course syllabus.

About five years ago, I decided that I wanted to answer the questions that I had been pondering all those years. To that end, I designed a qualitative phenomenological research study that focused on two key questions (see the "Research Overview" in appendix A):

- What significant career trajectory experiences on the executive path led to the CEO position?
- What key leadership competencies facilitated advancement on the executive path to CEO?

I wanted to explore these questions so that I could translate the lessons I learned into practical insights for racially and ethnically diverse professionals interested in pursuing the executive path and for the people supporting them in their careers. I also believed that other healthcare professionals and professors in health services administration would find the results useful, given the limited literature on this topic.

WHY DIVERSE CEOs?

While the other C-suite positions are important, and new roles continue to emerge as the healthcare landscape changes, I thought it would be informative to learn about the executive path to CEO specifically because of the need to increase diversity at that level. I have observed the significant impact that CEOs have on organizational culture, and studies have confirmed my observations. CEOs influence organizational culture by what they prioritize and act on, what they pay attention to, how they treat people, how they recognize people for their contributions, and how they use different leadership approaches to facilitate change and make everyday decisions. These are just a few examples of how top leaders, along with the senior executives they select and develop, have a strong impact on organizational culture. This impact permeates the organization, influencing leadership at all levels. I believe the lessons we learn from the racially and ethnically diverse executives in this book make a valuable contribution to the field.

Another important reason to look closely at diversity among healthcare executives is the changing demographics of the United States. The US population is becoming more racially and ethnically diverse, a fact that has been well documented in US Census Bureau projections and other population studies. Studies have linked this demographic change to the need for diverse leadership to enhance the cultural competence of healthcare organizations. As hospitals and health systems focus on developing healthy populations and

communities, the business case for increasing diversity in executive leadership becomes evident. Several studies that support this
thinking are cited in appendix A, "Research Overview."

SHARING WISDOM

I believe that racially and ethnically diverse professionals can
make a tremendous difference in healthcare organizations. I have
witnessed this time and again in my leadership and organization
development work and in my interactions with graduate students
in healthcare leadership. Yet textbooks and other resources rarely
highlight the experiences of racially and ethnically diverse leaders
or their leadership wisdom. We see more research and books written about private sector corporate executives than we do about
healthcare executives, particularly racially and ethnically diverse
professionals and women leaders. I want to help close this gap by
sharing what these individuals learned on the executive path and
how their leadership played a role in their advancement to the
C-suite.

LEADERSHIP DEVELOPMENT

I am passionate about leadership development and have worked in
the field for more than 30 years. As an African American woman
reflecting on my own career, especially early on, I realize now that
I did not have sufficient resources to help me navigate my career
journey. In some instances, I did not know how to access the
resources that were available at that time.

Later, as I advanced to higher-level positions, I was successful
in many ways, and yet I struggled because I lacked self-awareness
and an adequate circle of support. Mentors, coaches, and sponsors
were not recognized as essential for career advancement then, as
they are now, particularly for minorities and women. I did not

reach the executive level, for some of the reasons stated here. As I reflect on my career, I believe that what was most important to me was helping people make a difference and achieve the mission of the hospitals and health systems I worked in. I wanted to have greater access and capacity to do that. That meant more than having a vice president title.

The lessons learned from my experiences are another motivation for conducting this research and writing this book. While my passion for helping people has been, and remains, inclusive of all people, regardless of race, ethnicity, gender, sexual orientation, religion, and so on, as a black woman, I know that the path to executive leadership is harder. For this reason, I have a special interest in helping racially and ethnically diverse professionals avoid the mistakes I made and saw others make on their career journeys.

Another important point about leadership development for racially and ethnically diverse professionals is that we likely experience more challenges because of conscious and unconscious biases. I know I did, and I still do. For this reason, I want to provide a practical resource that has an implicit understanding of these challenges. More importantly, these challenges can be managed and overcome. The CEOs in this research study are good examples. Their experiences demonstrate that although racial/ethnic and gender biases exist, they need not be barriers to achievement.

THE BOOK

This book is based on research findings. It is about the lived experiences on the executive path of 12 racially and ethnically diverse hospital and health system CEOs. All but one of them were the CEO or top executive of a hospital or health system at the time of the interviews. The exception was a CEO who had transitioned to another executive position within the same health system by the time of the interview. The 12 executives include four African Americans, four Hispanic/Latino Americans, and four Asian Americans, with two men and two women in each group. The identities of these individuals and their organizations are kept confidential.

I would like to explain the use of the term "Hispanic" in this book. In the research study, the participants were identified as Hispanic, and they identified themselves in this manner. However, I am sensitive to the discussion, and sometimes debate, in the United States about the distinction between the terms "Latino" and "Hispanic." For example, two healthcare associations identify themselves differently: One is called the National Association of Hispanic Healthcare Executives, and the other is called the National Association of Latino Healthcare Executives. In this book, I will use the term "Hispanic/Latino" to respect both identifications.

This book is an opportunity to learn from the collective wisdom of all the executives. You will get a unique glimpse, from their perspectives, into what it takes to navigate the challenges and opportunities of the executive path to the C-suite.

Acknowledgments

THIS BOOK COULD not have been written without the generosity of the research study participants who willingly took time from busy schedules to share their stories, experiences, insights, and wisdom. I am sincerely grateful to each one of them, and I know the readers of this book are as well.

I want to express my gratitude to the Executive Commentators who supported this work by enthusiastically sharing their experiences and perspectives on individual chapters. Their comments added great value to this book.

The interest and encouragement of many people helped to make both the research and this book a reality. To all those who showed interest, shared suggestions, or gave words of encouragement, I express my heartfelt gratitude. I wish I could name all of them here; I regret that this space is limited.

There are a few people whom I would like to acknowledge here individually.

Fred Hobby, former president and CEO of the Institute for Diversity and Health Equity, was one of the first in the healthcare field to express an interest in this research. I emailed him in 2015 about my research idea and asked if he would be willing to have a brief telephone conversation with me to discuss it further. I was surprised how quickly he agreed, because we had never met and I was not well known in the field. I am very grateful for his ongoing, enthusiastic interest and encouragement.

Fred introduced me to Cynthia Washington, who was then director of member relations for the American Hospital Association (AHA) and later became interim president and CEO of the Institute for Diversity and Health Equity. Cynthia invited me to the AHA Diversity Roundtable meeting in May 2015. This invitation was significant because it gave me an opportunity to meet diverse healthcare executives and to begin discussing the research that I intended to conduct. I want to sincerely thank her for that important invitation and her continuing interest in this work.

One of the executives at that May 2015 meeting was Richard D. Cordova, FACHE, president emeritus of Children's Hospital Los Angeles. He expressed interest in the research and was open to me contacting him to discuss it further. I want to thank him for his generous encouragement and gracious support throughout this long journey.

It took another year of conversations to gain the courage to move forward with the research without external funding. In 2016 I contacted Cie Armstead, DBA, director of diversity and inclusion for the American College of Healthcare Executives (ACHE), to share my research idea. She was, and continues to be, an enthusiastic supporter whose encouragement throughout this journey has helped to sustain me. I thank her for her gracious support.

Cie introduced me to Leslie Athey, director of research for ACHE. I am grateful to Leslie for her interest and encouragement, which meant a great deal to me as I began to conduct the research.

I want to acknowledge and thank Luisa Franzini, PhD, professor and chair of the Department of Health Policy and Management at the University of Maryland School of Public Health. Signing the required approvals for the university's institutional review board helped make this research possible. I also thank Nedelina Tchangalova, the University of Maryland's public health librarian, for her invaluable assistance with literature searches.

Thanks are also due to Ray C. Rist, PhD, a qualitative research expert and a qualitative research methodology professor during my doctoral studies. Dr. Rist met with me several times to provide invaluable guidance on research methodology.

I could not have completed this work without my friends and circle of personal support. In particular, I want to express my deepest gratitude to Mary, a dear friend for many years, whose prayers and reassurance were much needed and helped me to get through this journey. I want to thank Sylvia, my forever friend since my days at Howard University, for her prayers, which always lift me up. I am so grateful to my dear friend Kathy, who has been listening to me and supporting me since I was 14 years old. I thank Father Joe, Ernie, Betty, Clare, and Gloria for listening and for their encouragement and prayers. I express my appreciation to Andrea, Rose Marie, and Betsy, whom I don't talk to often but who, when I do, always say "You can do it!" and cheer me on. I thank Trish, a good friend and colleague who has supported me enthusiastically from the beginning (and who told me I was writing a book before I could even begin thinking about it). Finally, I extend my sincere gratitude to Kathy at the yoga center and friends in the weekly meditation circle for helping me to quiet my mind and reduce stress.

I end these acknowledgments with accolades and respect for the professionalism and knowledge of the staff at Health Administration Press. Jennette McClain, acquisitions editor, recognized the value of this project in the first conversation I had with her. I cannot thank her enough for her guidance, honest feedback, support, and commitment to this book. Thank you to Andrew Baumann, editorial production manager, for guidance with the production process and for selecting a great manuscript editor. Sincere gratitude to Deborah Ring, an excellent manuscript editor, for her expertise and respect for my work. Thanks to Nancy Vitucci, marketing manager, for her marketing expertise. To the entire Health Administration Press team, I extend my sincere appreciation.

Introduction

ARE YOU INTERESTED in learning about the lived experiences of leaders on the executive path? Do you want to learn how racially and ethnically diverse healthcare CEOs achieved that level of leadership? Do you want to use the lessons learned from their experiences to navigate your own career journey? Are you a mentor, coach, sponsor, or healthcare professional who wants to better understand executive and leadership development and support diverse professionals? Are you a faculty member in a health services administration program, a public health program, or another healthcare leadership program who is interested in lessons on diverse leadership and career advancement for your graduate students?

Then this book is for you. You will learn from the collective wisdom of 12 racially and ethnically diverse CEOs who give insights into these questions. The stories they shared in interviews about their lived experiences on the executive path to the C-suite are filled with practical lessons.

INTERVIEWS REVEAL COMMON THEMES

This book is based on in-depth, face-to-face interviews with a group of 12 racially and ethnically diverse CEOs. Their identities and the names of the hospitals and health systems they work for remain confidential. At times, pseudonyms are used to protect their identities.

The interviews were conducted in two parts, totaling about three hours per executive. These meetings took place in the executive's office or in an adjacent meeting room. In most cases, I used the executive's résumé or curriculum vitae to learn about their executive path. The interviews began by asking about their background, including their parents, education, and people who influenced the early stages of their careers. Then, I asked about each position and job change on their career journey. Several key questions guided the inquiry in the first part of the interview protocol:

- What were your significant accomplishments? What did you learn from those accomplishments?
- What hardships (e.g., failures, mistakes, career setbacks) did you experience? How did you manage them? What did you learn from these experiences?
- What leadership competencies were gained from these experiences?
- What leadership competencies had the most significant impact on your advancement?
- What developmental relationships (e.g., mentors, sponsors, coaches) were particularly significant in your development as a leader?
- What developmental experiences had the most significant impact on you?

In the second part of the interview protocol, the following questions guided the inquiry:

- What impact has pursuing an executive path had on your family life?
- What do you do to maintain a balanced life?
- According to a 2015 study conducted by the Institute for Diversity in Health Management in collaboration with the Health Research and Educational Trust, only 9 percent

of CEOs belonged to racial/ethnic minority groups. Your career trajectory to CEO is still rare.

- – To what do you attribute your achievement as a minority?
- – In what ways do you think your experiences have been different from those of your white counterparts in healthcare administration?
- Has race/ethnicity created challenges in your career progression on the executive path? If so, how did you manage them? If not, why not?
- Has your race/ethnicity helped shape your leadership approach?

The analysis of the responses to these questions revealed several major themes, which are organized as the chapters in this book. Key insights and wisdom from the CEOs are shared in each chapter.

If you are looking for 10 or 12 steps to reach the C-suite, you will not find them in this book. I have learned that there is no set of quick steps to become a CEO. The executive path is not a step-wise upward ladder, but rather a journey that is filled with unpredictable twists and turns. You will learn that the executive path is a long and challenging journey that comprises complex learning and growth, accomplishments, setbacks, mistakes, and advancement in an uncertain healthcare environment. These executives did not experience perfect career trajectories, but their rich experiences ultimately led to the C-suite. Insights and lessons learned from them will help you navigate your own journey.

HOW THIS BOOK IS ORGANIZED

Each chapter in this book focuses on a theme that emerged from the interviews and includes practical experiences and stories that the CEOs shared. Each chapter ends with a summary of Key

Lessons. That summary is followed by an Executive Commentary section. This section includes perspectives from other diverse executives whom I interviewed about each theme, offering additional insights into and lessons about the executive path.

Finally, each chapter includes a Reflection and Action section, which provides an opportunity for you to reflect on your own experiences and learning and identify specific actions that you can take to advance your career and developmental relationships.

In chapter 10, "Discerning What Matters Most," I identify seven essentials for career development. Practicing these essentials will provide a foundation for your continuing growth and development as a person and as a leader. This chapter is intended to help you turn these essentials into practices that will make a difference in your career.

I end the book with thoughts and reflections on what I learned from the research and writing this book.

AN INVITATION

I invite you to make this book your own and to use whatever you learn to advance your career. Whatever your goal—whether it is to become a CEO, attain another C-suite leadership role, or reach an executive or nonexecutive position, or even if you are not sure what you want to do yet—my hope is that this book will help you decide how you will make a difference in healthcare. If you are a mentor, sponsor, coach, teacher, or other professional who supports the development of others, my hope is that this book will enrich your developmental relationships. Finally, for those of you who just want to learn more about diverse healthcare executives, I hope you find this book interesting.

CHAPTER 1

Backgrounds Are the Foundation

Do you think about your background and how it has influenced who you are today and how your career has progressed? As the executives interviewed for this research told their stories, all of them described how lessons learned from parents, family members, and other significant people in their lives remain with them today. Although the starting places for their careers were different, these executives shared many similarities with regard to the importance of education and a strong work ethic. This chapter explains what I learned about the enduring impact of background and how it is the foundation of an executive career.

EARLY LESSONS MADE A DIFFERENCE

Parents and relatives played the most significant role in developing the executives' early values about education and work. In each case, high expectations were set for education and achievement. Some of the executives' parents did not have much education themselves, yet they emphasized the importance of learning. For example, in one case, the executive's mother had a seventh-grade education and his father had completed the fifth grade. In this instance, the executive talked about how he had received support from his parents and learned from them the importance of education, the value of hard work, and the motivation to be better. Similarly, another executive's parents also had limited education, but his mother encouraged him to excel at school and gave him self-esteem. She did this by repeatedly telling him, "You can do it!" This is an example of how the early development of self-esteem and self-confidence can have an impact on an individual's career later in life.

Not every executive's parents had limited education. Some parents were educated and worked as professionals or business owners. In two cases, the entire family worked in healthcare and served as role models for attaining high levels of education and working in the healthcare field. Similarly, another executive's mother worked in healthcare. These parents inspired their children's early interest in the field.

Several executives came from families in which the parents were divorced, the father died, or there was a single-parent mother and an absent father. In a couple situations, grandmothers had a significant influence. For example, one executive talked endearingly about her grandmother, who encouraged her to go to college and to focus on a healthcare profession. She elaborated on how her grandmother taught her confidence and initiative to lead.

In addition to education, the executives learned valuable lessons about having a strong work ethic and doing their best. As one executive explained, her mother taught her to keep plugging along even during difficult times. The family was poor and lived in low-income housing. After her father died, her mother still managed to pay the bills and feed the family—an early lesson in perseverance. A key takeaway is that regardless of your family circumstances, it is possible to overcome them and learn positive values that will guide and sustain you throughout your life and career.

In one interview, a significant lesson emerged: "Being right . . . matters a lot less if you can't convince people of your position and if you can't figure out a middle ground with people that you disagree with." This executive learned an early lesson about finding common ground that he still values today. In another case, an executive talked about how both of her parents worked hard and remained loyal to the organizations in which they worked. Because of their example and the values they instilled in her, she knew that she would always work hard to achieve her goals and that loyalty is imperative.

Another significant lesson that most of the executives in the study shared was religious faith. Many talked about how their faith had sustained and guided them on their executive path. These executives described their faith as a moral compass. For example, one CEO explained, "This is what I believe: Until He is done with me, wherever He wants me, that's where I will be." Another said, "My version of true north is my faith and family." Still another executive said, "My view of this is all about a Higher Power ordering our steps and at times creating steps for us that we don't realize." For these leaders, faith was a source of strength and perseverance.

The lessons that these executives learned from their parents and family had a significant impact on their lives and careers. The roots of self-esteem and self-confidence began to take hold when they were young. Values such as loyalty, seeking common ground, perseverance, hard work, and doing their best developed as they pursued their careers. These values live on today as they carry out their executive roles. The high expectations that their families set led all of them to seek out graduate education.

GRADUATE EDUCATION WAS ESSENTIAL

The importance of education instilled by parents and family was evident in the fact that all the executives attained graduate degrees. All of them believed that graduate education played an essential role in their careers. It gave them a foundation of knowledge that proved valuable, especially at the beginning of their careers. Graduate education also helped them to be more competitive in the healthcare administration job market.

Among the executives studied, 6 out of 12 had earned a master of healthcare or health administration (MHA) degree. One executive earned a certificate in health services administration and a master of public administration degree. Another individual had both an MHA and a master of science in nursing. Three executives held a master of business administration (MBA) degree in addition to another graduate degree—a master's degree in health administration, a medical degree, or a master's degree in accountancy. One individual held a master of public health degree. Others held master of science and law degrees. While the MHA was predominant, based on the experience of these executives, other graduate degrees can be valuable for a healthcare administration career.

In most cases, the CEOs who had attained the MHA degree also participated in a postgraduate administrative fellowship or residency. These MHA programs linked top graduates to opportunities that would have been difficult to obtain on their own. The fellowships and residencies were essential stepping stones because they provided exposure to the executive level and valuable practical experiences in hospitals and health systems. After completion, the executives were offered positions with the host organizations. In these cases, fellowships and residencies accelerated advancement on the executive path. Those who did not have fellowships gained practical experience by attaining positions with the help of sponsors.

Graduate education was clearly necessary for career advancement in these cases. The combination of graduate education and early job experiences, which allowed the executives to demonstrate high performance and achievements, gave them an excellent start, although everyone did not come from the same functional background.

FUNCTIONAL BACKGROUNDS BROUGHT DIFFERENT PERSPECTIVES

The CEOs interviewed started from different functional backgrounds. They did not all begin in healthcare administration. Five had clinical backgrounds that included nursing, medicine, physical therapy, a physical therapy–related specialty, and medical technology. These individuals moved into leadership positions in their clinical areas and then progressed to hospital administration positions. As we will discuss in chapter 5, all of them had sponsors.

One executive worked as an attorney, and in that capacity he represented a hospital client. As a result of that relationship, he was offered a position as vice president of legal services for the hospital. This opportunity initiated his executive journey to CEO.

Another study participant began his career in industrial engineering and facilities management for a hospital. With additional graduate education, he worked his way into other operational positions. These experiences put him on the executive path, and later he was sponsored for a chief operating officer (COO) leadership development program. This program was the platform for his progression to his first hospital COO position.

As a result of their diversity of backgrounds, the executives brought different perspectives to the executive leadership role. It was not any easier for the executives with clinical and healthcare administration backgrounds to move along the executive path to CEO than it was for those who did not have such backgrounds. The key factor was sponsorship for positions that gave them experience, exposure, and opportunities to develop and to demonstrate their leadership capabilities. And, most importantly, they performed.

RESULTS WERE ACHIEVED THROUGH HIGH PERFORMANCE

The values that these executives learned from their parents and family led them to become high performers in school and during the early stages of their careers. In every case, the executives interviewed talked about the importance of making a difference. They all indicated that performance and results get noticed. As one said, "It is important to know what makes you stand out." He went on to say that it is important to ask, "What is going to make you significantly different than the other 100 résumés that are going to be submitted for the position you want?" Another said, "You have to perform and do the work; it's about people thinking that you're true to the mission and goals of the organization."

Many of the CEOs described how they had to work harder. One explained, "I had to earn my way in. If somebody gives 70 percent to be successful, I have to give 120 percent to be successful." He went on to say, "More is expected of me to earn where I am." Another revealed that he was willing to take on responsibility and challenges: "It was my work ethic."

The women interviewed made similar comments about their willingness to take on challenging assignments. They talked about how hard they had worked and how they had to do more than was expected of them. One said, "I worked a lot of nights. I got to see a whole different side of the hospital and how it operates." She attributed her success to her willingness to work hard and do more to learn. Another executive indicated that she always worked hard to achieve financial and quality outcome targets. Another talked about how she told her boss that she had the capacity to do more. She said, "Don't say yes to everything, and when you say yes, you must turn it in on time." Achieving phenomenal results and knowing the business, as one executive indicated, are essential to progression on the executive path, and that proved true for all these executives.

Additional examples of achieving high results included completing assignments ahead of schedule and on budget, implementing major capital projects such as building new hospitals, and turning organizations around to improve quality and financial results. As one of the women indicated, it is also important to communicate your results and achievements: You cannot assume that everyone in the organization, particularly the people who count, know what you are doing. You have to find ways to communicate your achievements and demonstrate how you are contributing to the organization's mission and shared goals. This needs to be done without arrogance and with humility, she went on to say. This important point represents the collective wisdom of all the executives interviewed.

BACKGROUNDS MATTER

For these executives, their backgrounds mattered because the lessons they learned well before their careers began provided a foundation for their executive path journeys. Self-esteem and self-confidence were instilled early. Values such as a keen work ethic, perseverance, loyalty, seeking common ground, education and learning, and faith made a difference in their lives and careers. Diverse functional qualifications and early job experiences in which they demonstrated high performance and achieved significant results were a foundation on which they built successful careers.

KEY LESSONS

- Values instilled early in life make a difference throughout your career and life journey.
- Graduate education is essential.
- Early experiences in fellowships, residencies, and internships can help launch your career.
- There is more than one way to get on the executive path.
- Where you start is important, but how you start—that is, living your positive values—is even more important.
  - Jobs and assignments that give you experience, exposure, and opportunities for leadership are imperative.
  - High performance, achieving results, and communicating achievements make a significant difference in how your potential is viewed.

EXECUTIVE COMMENTARY

"I think the influence about doing your best and believing in yourself comes from not only parents but also grandparents. My father taught me the power of positive thinking."

—Rick L. Stevens, FACHE, President,
Christian Hospital

"My mom was an environmental service cleaning lady at a hospital. I would visit her at work. She encouraged me to work there after graduating high school. I did the same job, cleaning rooms, and enjoyed connecting with the patients. Later I became a nurse technician. This is where my passion for patient care and helping others began. I wanted to see better care than my mom received. These early experiences are the foundation for my career in healthcare."

—Eddie Cruz, MBA, FACHE, Vice President of Operations,
Access Community Health Network

Reflection and Action

As you reflect on your own background,

- What is most significant for you?

- What gifts from your past can help you in your career today?

- What values were you taught that guide your life and work today?

- What are the roots of your self-esteem and self-confidence? What do you need to do to maintain them?

- What actions will you take to use the lessons and insights from your background to guide your career journey?

CHAPTER 2

Reflections on Race and Ethnicity

SINCE THE EXECUTIVES interviewed for this book are racially and ethnically diverse, I think it is important to share their reflections about race and ethnicity as it relates to their career journeys. In particular,

- Did race/ethnicity create any challenges on the executive path?
- What did these racially and ethnically diverse executives think about their advancement to the C-suite?

This chapter will answer these questions based on the interview responses. But first, I would like to clarify that the focus of this research and this book is not race/ethnicity. The focus is how racially and ethnically diverse professionals in hospitals and health systems achieved the CEO position. Simply put, how did they get to the C-suite, in light of the comparatively low percentage of diverse executives at this level? Specific open-ended questions about race and ethnicity were not asked until the second part of the interview protocol. However, the executives shared some comments about race and ethnicity as they told their stories in the first part of the interviews.

What about gender? Although gender was not the focus of this research, there were six women in the study. For this reason, it is important to recognize the "intersectionality" of race and gender (Crenshaw 1989). Intersectionality means that race and gender cannot be separated but are interconnected. This explains why the women often talked about their gender even though the questions focused on race and ethnicity.

What follows are the interview questions and the key themes that emerged from the responses. Quotations are used to illustrate the themes.

TO WHAT DO YOU ATTRIBUTE YOUR ACHIEVEMENT AS A MINORITY?

Hard Work and Performance

The study participants generally attributed their achievement to hard work and stellar performance:

- "I think . . . I do really good work. I work really hard. I do think some people have an entitlement problem. They think somebody owes them something. I think everything is a gift."
- "The sense that you have to be a cut above, got to be a little better, tends to make you work a little harder."
- "I do a lot of self-reflection—[for example,] Did I handle that meeting well? I've got this drive to do a better job of the work that I'm doing; not continuing to stay with status quo."
- "Hard work, being willing to get there and take chances; being willing to relocate; being willing to take on jobs you don't know; being willing to put in the hours to learn; being willing to listen and learn from others."

- "I work harder and think about how do I make sure my results are . . . pristine and . . . tiptop to develop credibility."
- "First and foremost, I have never thought of myself as a minority. But on the other side of the coin, I do know that I am a minority. I do know that there's racial tensions; there's bigotry; there is discrimination that exists in our world. I do know that I have to work a lot harder because I'm a person of color."
- "I really believe it's just your personal desire to be successful. You have to self-determine. As an immigrant, there is limitless opportunity to define yourself. You have to desire it to live a productive life."

Performance and hard work were the primary drivers of achievement for these executives. Underlying factors were their motivation to achieve and their perseverance.

Seeking Common Ground

The ability to appreciate the differences between racially and ethnically diverse professionals and their majority (white) colleagues in terms of their experiences and backgrounds, yet to seek common ground with them, was another theme. That is, rather than focusing on differences, these executives sought to find common ground with their colleagues to bridge gaps:

- "I literally think it is my ability to make them feel comfortable. They don't see me as threatening, aggressive, or whatever the stereotypes are. It really is challenging to get to a place where you feel like we have more in common than we don't. We tend to choose people that are like [ourselves], and that is the invisible barrier that we can't quite get through."

- "I had to learn to disarm people because of my ethnicity. The best way, 'common denominator.' If I walk into your office, within 30 seconds of being there, I have found something that you and I share in common."
- "I have the ability to function without giving up my identity as an African American in an industry dominated generally by Caucasian males."

Another study participant indicated that it is necessary to fit in and adapt to the organizational culture. A senior executive told this individual that to move up in the organization, they must fit a certain mold. In this case, the person was a high performer but was overweight and had to work on appearance. The other aspect of common ground is learning the common characteristics of successful executives in the organization and adapting to those qualities without losing identity and self-respect.

Mentors

It is no surprise that the executives consistently responded that mentors had contributed to their achievement:

- "I work hard but I still think it takes somebody nurturing you and positioning you."
- "I give credit back to my mentors. I sought them out. I had great mentors and sustained relationships [by] asking for feedback."
- "Mentors. I have a support system."
- "My experience of success is directly proportional to the mentorship and coaching that I got in my journey."

It is clear that having good mentors was significant for these executives' career trajectories. But sponsors also opened doors and provided opportunities for achievement.

Diverse Geographic Region or Organization

Several individuals indicated that living in a diverse geographic location or working in a diverse organization made race and ethnicity less of an issue in their career progression. One executive commented, "I have been successful in this part of the United States where theoretically my color, ethnicity, and race are commonplace." This person went on to say, "If you were to take me and say, 'You would be a great CEO in another geographic region,' I may not have the reception that I have had here." Likewise, another study participant stated, "I'm not a minority in this city." However, the executives underscored that being part of the majority race/ethnic group in a geographic location was not enough to facilitate advancement. What made the difference was hard work and accomplishments over the years.

In another case, an executive worked for a health system that was more diverse. She said, "I feel like that's always been a blessing, because in that setting, I have never been discriminated against. . . . I think I may have had a different experience otherwise." Similarly, a different person shared this perspective: "Both organizations that I worked for . . . were dedicated to looking at diversity within their workforces. When you have an organization that says 'That is important to us' and places diversity in its values, it is more open to diversity."

These perspectives suggest that levels of geographic and organizational diversity influence the experiences of racially and ethnically diverse professionals. One might posit that for executives who are not racial or ethnic minorities in these contexts, their race or ethnicity presents less of a barrier to career advancement. Of course, more evidence is needed to substantiate that hypothesis.

Positive Outlook

An underlying theme in all of the executives' responses is that a positive outlook contributed to their achievement. They did not focus on their race or ethnicity. While these executives were conscious of their race and did not lose their identities, they did not let race or ethnicity distract them from their mission to become effective leaders in healthcare. They did not view all of their experiences through a racial or ethnic lens, which could have led them to become preoccupied with it. As one executive said, "I don't get caught up in why I'm different." They directed their energy and attention to service and making a difference. Their intention to succeed transcended any negativity that they faced on their career journeys.

The key factors that contributed to the achievement of these racially and ethnically diverse executives are woven throughout this book. Their responses give us additional insights into their thinking on race and ethnicity.

IN WHAT WAYS DO YOU THINK YOUR EXPERIENCES HAVE BEEN DIFFERENT FROM THOSE OF YOUR WHITE COUNTERPARTS?

Many of the executives expressed a belief that as racial/ethnic minorities, they had to work harder. One executive said, "The white counterpart climbed the ladder much faster," but noted, "I work twice as hard in some regards." Another individual indicated, "I believe and know that I have to work harder and do more to just be in the same place." This person continued, "There is a sense of privilege that comes with being a majority leader. . . . As a minority, I don't have that perspective of privilege; I'm working at it." Similarly, this individual said, "I sometimes think there is less to prove on their part than there is on mine." Another person concurred with this perspective: "I have to earn my way in. More is expected of me to earn where I am."

Many, but not all, of the executives also expressed that some of their white colleagues had different assumptions about them or lower expectations of them because of their race/ethnicity. An individual shared, "I don't think there were a lot of assumptions that I was going to be able to accomplish whatever I have been able to accomplish. I was always kind of comfortable with that. It's a reality that you have to accept. At this career juncture, people look at my track record." Another executive revealed, "What they would see in me, the same characteristics in a white person, where I was seen as arrogant and cocky, he was seen as competent and professional."

This seemed to be a common understanding, and it was accepted as a given for most of the executives interviewed. But their acceptance was not angry or negative. Rather, they accepted the reality and were not preoccupied with it. Know who you are and achieve—that is what they did by exceeding expectations.

Another insight from the executives was that their white counterparts, because of their majority status and the forces of structural racism, may have had experiences that some racially and ethnically diverse professionals have not had—golfing and playing tennis at country clubs, boating, formal black-tie dinners, and other elite social events. The lack of exposure to these types of experiences can create barriers for career advancement. As we have learned, so much of developing meaningful business relationships happens in social settings. How one dresses, behaves, and interacts with others are often unspoken criteria for advancement. Several executives interviewed for this study noted, particularly early in their careers, learning to play golf, getting advice on appropriate attire and behavior at formal events, and participating in training on communication and media skills. They learned to adapt and fit in, not only with the organizational cultures in which they worked but also with the social cultures in which they found themselves.

The differences that some participants expressed may be related to negative assumptions and low expectations of racially and ethnically diverse professionals that are rooted in stereotypes. They are not always spoken but can subtly undermine achievement and opportunities. The belief that minorities cannot perform or are not suitable for leadership can fuel implicit biases. As a result of these biases, racially and ethnically diverse professionals may not be selected for high-visibility assignments that lead to promotion. The executives in the study did not focus on these issues, but rather on the high performance needed to achieve the organizational goals associated with their positions. Also, they learned early on that it was important for them to actively participate in different types of organizational and social events. They understood the value of informal networking and letting people get to know them to develop meaningful relationships.

HAS RACE/ETHNICITY CREATED CHALLENGES IN YOUR CAREER PROGRESSION ON THE EXECUTIVE PATH?

Gender More Than Race

Several executives in the study rejected the idea that their race/ethnicity had created challenges in their career progression. Two of them were women who believed that their gender was more of an issue. In one case, the executive was told directly that a certain region in the health system was not ready for a female CEO. She reflected, "It has been gender that has created challenges on the executive path." Further, she stated, "I was never exposed to being treated differently because of my ethnicity, probably because I grew up in a minority community." On one occasion in her first top executive position outside of that community, a board member asked the executive "what tribe she was from." The same question was asked of another female CEO study participant. Both women expressed that they did not take the incidents personally and used them as teaching moments to explain that they were not from a tribe. They used them as opportunities to educate others about who they are.

Another female executive expressed that gender was revealed as an issue early in her career, when she felt like an outsider working in a male-dominated executive team. It was important for her to overcome this feeling so that her voice could be heard at the table. She reflected, "I started thinking, 'I have to sit at the table and have that presence,'" referring to her executive demeanor. In doing so, she found her voice and began sharing her perspectives and gaining respect from the team.

Did Not Present Challenges

Four other executives did not believe that their race or ethnicity had presented challenges for them—at least not in ways that influenced their career trajectories. In the first case, the executive expressed that he was not a minority in the city where he lived, and because of that, he believed he did not experience racism. He said that minorities need to understand that they will face challenges related to race and ethnicity because the culture of America is primarily white. He made two suggestions: Try not to get pigeonholed into certain jobs because of race or ethnicity, and let white people get to know you so that they can learn who you are, thereby minimizing stereotypes.

In the second case, the executive indicated that her initial goal was not to become a CEO. She did not push it. In her case, opportunities emerged because of her performance and her ability to work well with people and build teams. This person worked for a very diverse organization.

In the third case, the executive revealed that she could not think of any specific instances when her race had created a challenge for her advancement. This did not mean that she had never experienced racial microaggressions, however. Microaggressions are defined as "brief and commonplace daily verbal, behavioral, or environmental indignities, whether intentional or unintentional, that communicate hostile, derogatory, or negative racial slights and insults toward people of color" (Sue et al. 2007, 271). She pointed out that if she focused on criticisms and incidents, whether subtle or not, related to her race and gender, that would be a distraction. Her decision was to focus on excellence.

Finally, in the fourth case, the executive did not mention racial challenges as barriers to advancement. He did talk, however, about being the one who worked the hardest, coming in early and leaving late and doing work that many other people were not doing. In describing one situation, he reflected, "Part of it was that I'm the only person of color in this place. If I'm not better, then I'm not even equal." This awareness was implied throughout the interviews, but it did not become a preoccupation, and this executive felt that he did not lose his identity. Again, the focus was on performance and service. He learned to work effectively in the white male–dominated healthcare industry.

Presented Challenges

In the six other cases, the executives believed that race and ethnicity had created challenges in some situations. One executive described these challenges as "linked to breaking down the stereotypes or perceptions that others have about how you are supposed to behave or what you are supposed to be like." For example, in the hospital where this executive worked, the majority of the physicians were white men over 50 who liked sports, golf, whiskey, and flying. She did not share most of these interests. She said, "Here's the challenge as a minority woman—how to build a relationship with them and find a connection." Her solution was to talk about what they did have in common and their mutual interests. She gave another example from her career before she reached the C-suite, when there were no people of color on the leadership team. The organization was slow to promote her. Reflecting on whether race played a role, she said, "I try not to focus on it, frankly. . . . I'd like to think that my accomplishments should speak louder than anything else, and if my diverse opinion adds value, great."

In another case, an executive revealed that he had experienced discrimination. He said, "I have seen bigotry in the workplace and personally." He went on, "You have to face that and you have to act on it, if it is actionable. You have to have courageous leadership to lead through it with the purpose of making the environment that you are in better."

Another study participant responded in this way: "More often than not you are in a room where you are one or one of a very few. The more you are in a situation where the majority is unlike you, the more . . . potential challenges you face because of ignorance and lack of knowledge." When asked how he had navigated that situation, he responded, "By performing in [the] mainstream and constantly trying to tear the walls down."

In this case, the executive believed at one point in his career that he was being pigeonholed in a particular market because of his ethnicity. In other positions, he had experienced racist comments. For example, in one instance, a white male CEO openly made stereotypical comments about Spanish culture. On another occasion, a white male senior executive made negative remarks about different races, religious groups, and gay people. The study participant indicated that he managed these racial dynamics by working around them, not letting the remarks interfere with doing his job, and at times deflecting. He believed that his determination and focus on learning in those positions helped him manage these dynamics and achieve at a high level.

In another case, the executive said that she did not think about race or ethnicity early in her career. She had known some people who believed they had been discriminated against, but she never had those feelings. Reflecting on her career in the interview, she responded, "Now that I look back, 40 years later, I realize being diverse really did impact me. . . . I guess when I look back there were cues. I didn't listen to them—didn't know what they meant, or I was so positive that I would tune out anything negative." She continued by indicating that "part of the skill of an executive is really to tune out certain things." Further, she said, "Successful people never sit on their negatives; don't stew over it."

When asked whether race or ethnicity had presented a challenge, another executive responded, "I'm sure it has." He expressed that all people come to every situation with inherent biases and perspectives. Reflecting on his career, he indicated that people make certain assumptions about him. He continued, "I don't know if you ever in your personal and professional life overcome these. What I think I have done is accepted that as part of my reality and not let it define me. But never make the mistake of believing that it is not there. You accept a certain reality and move people past it with your performance."

In summary, the study participants' responses suggest that by focusing on performance and achieving career milestones with courage and perseverance, they were able to navigate any challenges related to their race/ethnicity or gender.

HAS YOUR RACE/ETHNICITY HELPED SHAPE YOUR LEADERSHIP APPROACH?

In all but one case, the executives in the study believed that their race or ethnicity had helped shape their leadership. The exception was an executive who indicated that being a minority had not shaped his leadership approach, but rather had helped him be more sensitive to issues. The following are some of their comments on this question:

- "Absolutely—because of my race, I also want to be an example. I want everybody to say, 'Here is somebody I would like to learn from.'"
- "My life experience, of which my ethnicity is a part . . . has shaped my leadership approach. I believe my style is one that is collaborative. I try not to enter into certain

assumptions when I meet people. I try not to bring to the table what I think many bring to the table with me."

- "I clearly believe more in collaboration and embracing difference than maybe some of my counterparts. . . . Issues around health equity and health disparities are important to me. I think discussing social impacts and social determinants of health are as important as how . . . we get our operating margin targets."

- "Oh yes, absolutely. . . . My race, because of being Asian, it's more communal. . . . Leadership emanated from how I was raised."

- "It has, humility. . . . I tell the team, 'Never hesitate to tell me when you think something is wrong.'"

- "The ability to be able to recognize there are differences in people and to be more sensitive. We need to not only respect that, we need to seek that out."

- "Absolutely—I think it is very clear that I lead with my heart. . . . Being an African American female probably gives me a little bit more sensitivity around various issues."

- "Probably in some way culturally. I am not obsessed with being perceived as being in charge, being the boss. I think that has assisted in shaping my management style. I am all about the team."

- "I think it helps me listen to dissent a little bit better, and listen to the quiet voice in the room who may not be speaking up. Active listening cannot be underestimated. . . . I think also integrity, I truly mean knowing where your limits are; knowing your push points; knowing these are the boundaries I don't cross; being values driven."

- "I'm sure it does. If you look at Hispanic culture, it is based on extended family. But it is not fair to say that because there are a lot of cultures that have a focus on family. But I think when you have a . . . strong cultural foundation that has certain values, I think you absolutely carry that through your leadership style."

- "Oh yes, significantly. The inability of my parents to access care as poor minorities has helped me make a lot of my value decisions as a leader. I want every patient to have the same experience that I want for my family whether they are rich or poor, black, white, brown, or green. I want them to have the same experience as anybody else."

These executives shared a belief that who they are as racial/ethnic minorities or as women helped shape them as leaders. They had a greater sensitivity to what it is like to be different or the only one in the room. With that sensitivity, they were able to be more inclusive. Collaboration and teamwork were consistent and interrelated leadership approaches that were influenced by this sensitivity. As one person said, "My ethnicity is part of my life experience . . . my life experience has shaped my leadership approach." The implication is that you cannot separate race and ethnicity or gender from your leadership approach.

Many important lessons can be gleaned from the study participants' reflections on navigating race and ethnicity on the executive path. At the core of these lessons is the intention to do the best work in service to mission. To promote health and to provide the highest-quality healthcare to individuals and communities in a culturally competent manner was central to their work. That was the driving purpose in their executive path journey.

The reality in the United States and elsewhere is that racially and ethnically diverse professionals are still often treated differently than their white counterparts and have a harder time achieving senior-level positions in healthcare. A gap persists between the increasingly diverse demographics of the people served by healthcare organizations and the C-suites of hospitals and health systems. However, executives who achieved this level of leadership expressed that it can be done with dignity, determination, and resilience.

KEY LESSONS

- Maintain identity, self-respect, and self-esteem.
- Hard work and high performance contribute to achievement.
- Focus on purpose and excellence.
- Discover what you have in common with colleagues of all racial/ethnic groups and genders.
- Broaden your comfort zone: Participate in social events and informal networking with people who are different from you.
- A positive outlook helps transcend biases and barriers.
- Manage microaggressions with dignity and use them as teaching moments.
- Do not focus on negative assumptions and lower expectations based on racial/ethnic or gender stereotypes.
- Embrace who you are and how your identity influences your leadership.

EXECUTIVE COMMENTARY

"Sometimes successful minorities in leadership positions early [in their] careers can experience some 'haterism.' This means people putting you down because of your success, particularly in organizational cultures that are not effectively working on diversity and inclusion. I think at some point you have to come to terms with that possibility and not let it get in the way of your success."

—Dr. Sachin H. Jain, MD, MBA, President and CEO, CareMore Health

"As an Asian American woman, I knew early in my career that the combination of my passion to contribute and impact communities, along with my dedication to having a good work product, would give me an opportunity to be competitive in healthcare management. I mentally dedicated myself to that because I knew I had multiple factors working as an obstacle. As a result, I have succeeded based on my own merit."

"Reflecting later in my career from a race, gender, and age perspective, I think authenticity and remaining genuine with yourself are really important. It's a balance to figure out how to keep your culture alive and how to assimilate or adapt so that you are accepted."

—Coleen Santa Ana, President, Sentara Albemarle Medical Center

"I would like to think that my talent in every aspect of my career has contributed to my success. Authenticity and awareness have helped me as a woman of color. Who I am has been a strength. My race and gender have influenced my leadership approach in that I strive to give everyone a voice and work to create an inclusive environment."

—Denise Brooks-Williams, Senior Vice President and CEO, North Market, Henry Ford Health System

REFERENCES

Crenshaw, K. 1989. "Demarginalizing the Intersection of Race and Sex: A Black Feminist Critique of Antidiscrimination Doctrine, Feminist Theory, and Antiracist Politics." *University of Chicago Legal Forum* 140: 139–67.

Sue, D. W., C. M. Capodilupo, G. C. Torino, J. M. Bucceri, A. M. B. Holder, K. L. Nadal, and M. Esquilin. 2007. "Racial Microaggressions in Everyday Life: Implications for Clinical Practice." *American Psychologist* 62 (4): 271–86.

CHAPTER 3

Positive Personal Qualities

When was the last time you thought about the person within you—that is, your positive personal qualities? Can you identify the qualities that have helped you along your career journey? This chapter reveals the positive personal qualities that influenced the career trajectories of the executives interviewed for this study.

THE VALUE OF THE PERSON WITHIN

Positive personal qualities influenced how the executives navigated their career journeys. These qualities are mirrors to the "person within." The person within is the compass that helped these executives manage their career trajectories. Positive personal qualities emerged early in their lives and were rooted in their backgrounds. These qualities transcend the executive path. As the study participants described their jobs and life experiences, it became clear that several distinguishing qualities defined them. Positive personal qualities influenced their frame of mind and their approach to life and work. They acted as guideposts that both grounded and elevated them in the midst of the complex day-to-day challenges they faced in hospitals and health systems.

In each case, the manner in which the executives managed their positions and situations demonstrated how their positive personal qualities enabled them to make significant career choices. They had several key qualities in common. As you read their stories, reflect on your own positive personal qualities and think about how they influence your thoughts, your mindset, your behavior, and your decisions along your career journey.

POSITIVE PERSONAL QUALITIES

What qualities had the most impact on these executives' career advancement? This is not just a list of good qualities. These qualities are positive characteristics that were significant because of the way the executives embodied and applied them. They are interrelated, working together to define each individual as a person and as a leader. As one executive said, "I sharpened awareness of self, tools, and insights to know myself and [to] know the personal side that would contribute to the professional side." While other qualities were discussed as the stories unfolded, those described here had the greatest impact on navigating the executive path.

Self-Awareness

The ability to know and understand oneself is vital for advancement in life and work. Reflecting on essential questions—Who am I? What do I need to do to become a better person and a better leader?—proved to be invaluable for the executives in this study. These professionals developed self-awareness early in their lives and maintained it throughout their careers. One study participant said, "I knew early on [that] making money was not my big motivator. I wanted to make a difference. I've always been a person [for whom] my personal values . . . [have] to be attuned with what I do. They have to be consistent with who I am."

Another reflected on an early experience and acknowledged, "In my mentality as a 20-plus-year-old, I probably did not have good emotional intelligence at the time." He acknowledged that not having well-developed emotional intelligence early in his career affected his decision-making and choices.

In another case, an executive disclosed, "I realized that sometimes I had to be less of me and more of what the situation required." He had to reflect deeply to become aware of the behaviors that he needed to adapt in a particular situation and why.

Yet another said, "I like to think I am pretty self-aware, so I know my shortcomings. I am learning to accept what I am very strong at and . . . [I am] comfortable saying that I am strong at those things." While talking about the decision to become a CEO, a different executive asked, "I know who I am, but who am I going to become?"

The others interviewed shared similar reflections. They recognized the critical importance of looking honestly at themselves in different situations and understanding their strengths and opportunities for growth. Mentors, coaches, and sponsors as well as colleagues, friends, and significant others helped them develop self-awareness through observations and constructive feedback.

Self-awareness was also linked to self-confidence in the interview responses. As these executives worked on developing self-awareness throughout their career journeys, they gained trust in their ability to lead and to succeed.

Values

The role that values play in life and career decision-making is related to self-awareness. Values are an individual's principles or standards of behavior, which reflect their judgments about what is important in life. The executives interviewed were values centered. One executive stated, "Whatever you do in your career, you have got to live out your life with your value system in place and solid."

Another believed, "Never compromise your character. Be true to who you are and be of good values. Your character defines [you]." A related comment supports this thinking: "Acknowledge when you are not correct." The ability to admit mistakes is character in action.

Values were also evident as the executives talked about their choice to pursue a career in healthcare. Their comments were aligned with their passion for providing high-quality healthcare. One person discussed the importance of "doing what you love." Another talked about the significance of "doing things for the right reasons rather than the money." In all cases, the executives were patient centered. They made comments such as "Do what is best for the patient" and "Have an unrelenting focus on the patient." They spoke about wanting to make a difference in the lives of the people they served. One executive explained what many of the leaders expressed in different ways: "I'm a steward of someone's investment, be it public with this hospital or a private facility with any of the for-profits. This is on loan to us to manage. We have a responsibility to that entity to do right." In each case, the executives interviewed stayed connected to the purpose of person-centered care. As one said, "When faced with the unknown, do what is best for the patient."

Together, having self-awareness and being values centered worked together to guide these executives on their career paths.

Integrity

Integrity is a quality that manifests from the inside out, like self-awareness and values. It is a quality that, on the surface, may seem easy to define. However, leading with integrity is difficult amid constant demands that test the ability to act on it routinely. Integrity is acting with internal consistency guided by moral principles and honesty. In business language, integrity has often been described as "walking the talk" or doing what you say you are going to do. Another common expression is "actions speak louder than words." That was true for these leaders.

In every case, the executives interviewed described situations that tested their integrity. It was apparent that their decisions were guided by consistent principles and values. Integrity requires not only articulating values and principles but also acting on them amid complex and sometimes conflicting demands. The executives shared stories filled with examples of integrity in action:

- "[I] always [acted] with honesty and strong integrity; I always told the truth."
- Sharing a story about raising children as a single parent and at the same time working with a hospital that was being investigated: "It was really hard. . . . It was a test of character. . . . I knew my integrity was solid. . . . I was going to stick with it."
- Recounting a difficult situation: "You focused on the vision and goals; open, honest conversation; acting with integrity; and not getting caught up in the messiness."
- Reflecting on gaining respect and acting with integrity: "I think over time when people see that you are purposeful, driven, fair, and try to do the right thing."

These examples demonstrate the significance of integrity as an enduring quality that informed these executives' leadership and influenced their career advancement.

Positive Outlook

It is well understood that an individual's general attitude toward life and work affects behavior and outcomes. Throughout the interviews, it was apparent that all of the executives had a positive outlook on life and on their careers. A positive outlook does not mean looking at the world through rose-colored glasses or failing to see the hard realities of healthcare leadership. For these leaders, it meant having a mindset that allowed them to see possibilities in the midst of complex challenges.

All of the executives expressed the attitude that they could manage tough situations and overcome barriers. This did not mean ignoring the negatives, however, and sometimes they expressed how difficult it was to endure some of their experiences. Tough experiences included taking over complicated organizational situations, following unsuccessful leaders, making changes in senior leadership approaches, managing bad leadership, and leading mergers and acquisitions. Belief in themselves and their ability to develop teams and the teamwork required to deal with challenging situations and achieve organizational goals set them apart from those who were stymied by such experiences:

- "I think everything in life is all about attitude."
- "I look at things in a positive [way]."
- "Making sure that I remained positive was very important."

This positive outlook shared by the executives was both influential and sustaining. It was influential in that it shaped the way they approached their careers and leadership. It was sustaining in that a positive outlook helped them endure particularly tough times. A positive outlook also gave them confidence that they could do the work and lead effectively. A positive outlook was a significant factor in all of the executives' career trajectories.

Work Ethic

A defining characteristic of all the executives was that they were hardworking and had a strong work ethic that fueled their passion for healthcare. The participants talked about this quality in a variety of ways. When asked about the factors that contributed to their success, the executives consistently identified work ethic—that is, the enduring belief that hard work is a value that drives success:

- "I was very organized, very diligent, and hardworking."
- "[I was] a hard worker wanting to do better."
- "It's about staying driven; you can't do the job without a drive; [it is] not so much about intellect as it is will."
- "I think I worked harder than the other two [colleagues], to be honest."

One executive described a conversation she had with her boss early in her career. She told him, "I want you to know that I have more time to do more. . . . I want you to know that I have the capacity to work on that." The result was a promotion. The willingness to do more than expected was a common theme in this study.

In all of the interviews, the executives identified a strong work ethic and hard work as the driving forces behind their high achievement.

Initiative

Another quality that helped these executives stand out on their career paths was initiative: taking the initiative to learn and do more than was required of them. In all cases, the study participants described themselves as people who did not wait for opportunities but had the vision to see them as they were developing. As one executive said, "Everyone is smart and had advanced degrees. The only thing that sets you apart is initiative."

Likewise, another executive spoke of the importance of developing the qualities that make you different from other competent people. Just being competent is not enough. This executive also talked about volunteering to follow up on projects that had been discussed in a meeting early in her career. For example, she would say, "I'll take a stab at doing it. Let me draft something and you can take a look at it." She confided that there were times when she did not know how to do the task she had volunteered for, but she was willing to take a risk. That strategy paid off: She received promotions and was a valued team member.

In that case, the executive worked beyond her normal work hours. She went to work in a different department to learn about its responsibilities. She socialized with colleagues who had skills and know-how that she wanted to learn. She took the initiative to identify these people and developed relationships with them. Again, the payoff was advancement to positions with increased responsibility.

A different executive revealed, "I had an innate curiosity that drove me to figure it out. . . . I didn't wait for someone to call me in to say, 'Let me show you how to do this.'" Another executive commented, "They loved that I was curious and always asking questions." Yet another person shared an important lesson: "I presented myself as somebody who was willing to take on responsibility and challenges."

As these comments indicate, taking initiative helped these executives stand out from their colleagues and proved to be a key factor in their career advancement. In these cases, the executives took initiative in a noncompetitive manner. In other words, they were not trying to beat their colleagues; rather, they were sincerely curious, hardworking, and wanted to learn and grow. These executives viewed their colleagues as team members and, in many instances, sources of learning and meaningful relationships.

Willingness to Take Risks

Sometimes taking initiative involves the willingness to take risks. Risk implies that something may not work out as intended or, worse yet, fail. The willingness to take risks on the executive path is a quality that all the executives had in common. They took assignments and positions that involved risk. In many cases, they managed difficult situations that involved organizational change.

In addition, all the executives interviewed were given "stretch" assignments that involved work they had not done before. Such assignments provide leadership development in action by giving leaders the chance to do new work, lead new teams, take on broader horizontal and vertical responsibility, and make operational and strategic decisions. Here is what one executive said about taking on this type of assignment: "It was sort of a stretch. . . . Even the recruiter who contacted me said, 'It's a stretch, but let's give it a shot and see.'" The executive went on to say, "Anytime you have a job that does not scare you, it's probably not much of a job." This opportunity for executive leadership was in a much larger hospital that was part of a growing health system. It facilitated his career advancement.

In a different case, an executive who took on a new assignment reflected, "We will figure it out." This indicated this individual's confidence in taking on the assignment and recognition that there were aspects of it that would require risk and new learning. Another person revealed, "It was a big risk because I'm leaving a pretty senior operations position." In describing this move, the executive said, "My career has always been [made up of] these opportunities to do something that I have not done before."

The willingness to take risks proved to be a critical quality for these executives. Each move on the executive path had inherent risk. In fact, one of the interviewees indicated that risk is inherent in executive and C-suite positions. Those who are interested in pursuing this level of leadership, she indicated, must not only accept this fact but also prepare themselves to manage risk. With higher risk comes more opportunity for mistakes and failure. A foundation of self-awareness, values, integrity, and positive outlook, along with an openness to learning, were essential qualities that enabled these leaders to be risk takers. These qualities need continuous development on the journey of life and leadership.

Openness to Learning

The executives interviewed used the phrase "I learned" many times. Each one was open to learning, seizing every opportunity to gain new skills, competencies, and experiences. They also applied what they had learned from previous experiences. One of them said, "I just really tried to soak up everything I could." The other executives expressed the same openness to learning:

- "It's being able to learn and understand what processes work and what [don't]."
- "Learn what you can: Taking opportunities to 'build my toolkit' was critical for advancement."
- "In new situations in which you have no or limited experience, learn—don't panic."

The value of listening was also discussed as an essential aspect of learning. It is important to note that most of these executives' learning took place in action, while they were engrossed in their work. These executives had an attitude that all they did and continued to do was about learning—accomplishments, successes, mistakes, failures, and regrets.

In addition to learning in action, several of the study participants went back to school because they recognized that they needed certain knowledge and skills to progress on the executive path. One of the executives made this point in talking about his early career: "I had to tool myself—because one of the deficits in my academic training was not taking accounting, finance, business, or law classes, all of which were key to my job. . . . So every chance I got I would find a workshop or seminar, basic accounting in business, finance in healthcare. It was self-development." Similarly, in other cases, the executives either pursued additional graduate degrees or engaged in other formal education to obtain knowledge and skills critical for their career advancement.

Required learning for executive leadership positions is continuously changing as the industry changes. It is essential to keep up-to-date on the knowledge, skills, and abilities that are required for leadership in healthcare. Openness to learning in action and continuing to learn in different ways are common characteristics that facilitated leadership development and progression on the executive path.

Adaptability

The ability to adapt to the changing healthcare environment is another important quality that the executives shared. They adapted their behaviors, actions, and leadership approaches to work effectively in different organizational cultures. These executives transitioned in and out of organizations and situations throughout their careers. Transitioning and adapting are ongoing.

One executive defined adaptability this way: "It is about being observant and adaptable to the circumstances you are in." Another executive reflected, "I shifted gears and stopped my service line activity at the hospital and moved to open a clinic." In each case, the CEOs studied were continuously navigating change and adapting. Self-awareness and assessment of the situation are evident in all the stories.

Adaptability does not mean changing who you are in different situations, as the executives pointed out. It is disingenuous to shift who you are like a chameleon. These leaders were genuine, and that is why they were respected. The ability to adapt effectively calls on self-awareness, values clarification, integrity, and openness to learning new ideas and new ways of doing things in moments of leadership action.

The executives told stories about competing values and conflicts between what was expected and what they believed to be the most appropriate direction at the time. They were mindful of how much they would adapt, guided by their strong sense of integrity and values. Adaptability is a balancing and discernment process. In the real world of leadership, things are not often "either-or" situations. So much of leadership in healthcare is about working collaboratively to reach common ground and frequently compromising or accommodating without losing your identity and purpose. These executives demonstrated adaptability time and again, validating adaptability as an invaluable quality for advancement.

Humility

An interesting observation made by each executive was the level of humility that leadership requires. It was obvious during the interviews that they were not preoccupied with status or power in a negative sense. The language they used to describe themselves and their experiences was not boastful. Most of the executives interviewed used the term "humility" to describe their leadership approach. When asked about their accomplishments, they made statements such as the following:

- "It draws on your humility."
- "I think a lot of it is humility."
- "Be in a place of humility."
- "There is this balance of humility and confidence."
- "I always approach it as a humble experience. . . . I always say develop a sense of humility."
- "Never taking yourself that serious, at the same time knowing there is a purpose and reason for why you are doing what you are doing."

One executive summed up humility this way: "When we develop so much hubris around our titles [and] successes, life at times has an interesting way of bringing you back to earth when you think you are too smart and you've gotten beyond things. I always say develop a sense of humility. I always try to make the . . . successes not be about me and make it about other people." These comments give us insight into the quality of humility possessed by the executives in this study.

Perseverance and Resilience

Perseverance and resilience go hand in hand. To persevere in the face of difficult situations is to keep striving for excellence and doing your best work in service to the healthcare mission. Resilience is the ability to bounce back from difficulties, such as disappointments, mistakes, and setbacks. The executive path is filled with twists and turns, ups and downs. The executives cited real-world examples of difficulties they had encountered during their careers: being fired for political reasons, even when organizational goals were accomplished; positions not working out because they were not a good fit; being falsely accused; or senior colleagues suggesting there was a trust issue without facts to support the assertion. In every case, perseverance and resilience allowed the executives to learn, grow, and rise above the challenges.

As one of the executives said, "I'm someone who is resilient and not focused on the negatives." Another talked about the importance of "learning to deal with adversity" and not letting adversity define you as a leader. In a different case, perseverance was described this way: "It's persistence; not blind persistence but when you get on the path and you know for sure it's the right path, even when the big boulders get thrown in the middle of the way, you stay true to the path." As these words and examples teach us, resilience is essential to navigating the tough terrain of the executive path. It is the ability to maintain emotional and psychological hardiness in the midst of adversity. It is not being taken down by difficult times but working through them to recover and move forward stronger as a result of experience. That is what these executives did well.

The interrelationships among these positive personal qualities are apparent. These qualities do not operate in isolation or in a linear manner. They work together to define the person within (see exhibit 3.1). In addition, while faith is not a quality per se, as discussed in chapter 1, most of the interviewees talked about their faith as a moral compass that was ingrained in them. The qualities that define the person within act as navigational aids on the executive path.

EXHIBIT 3.1: Interrelationships Among Positive Personal Qualities

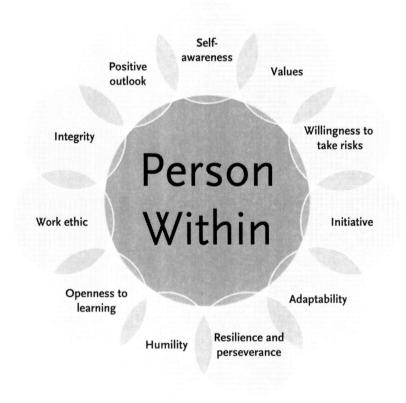

KEY LESSONS

- Personal qualities define the "person within."
- Gaining awareness of the person within requires working from the inside out to become mindful and self-aware.
- Positive personal qualities are interrelated. It is important to understand how they work together to develop the person within.
- Understanding how personal qualities affect behavior and decision-making is essential for leadership development.
- Positive personal qualities play a key role in becoming an effective person and leader.
- Being centered in positive values and personal qualities helps guide and sustain balance during challenging times.
- Positive personal qualities influence success on the executive path.

EXECUTIVE COMMENTARY

"There are several qualities that have influenced my advancement. I think perseverance has had a big effect. I define perseverance as not giving up and going on with your dream and goal. Another quality is flexibility, particularly the willingness to move geographically for career advancement. Fortunately, I have a spouse that has that flexibility as well. The other quality is integrity. Your integrity is a big piece of who you are and it follows you everywhere you go. An additional quality that guides my career trajectory is faith. For me, that means faith in God and yourself, trusting that everything is going to work out."

—Rick L. Stevens, FACHE, President, Christian Hospital

"I generally find myself in an environment where I am likely the only or the other. I believe you have to get used to being uncomfortable and stay focused on creating alignment among others through driving the mission and a positive outlook to drive performance. That is more important than physical differences."

—Coleen Santa Ana, President,
Sentara Albemarle Medical Center

"I think first and foremost my honesty and integrity are qualities that people respect and have helped me to succeed as a healthcare executive."

"Another quality that has made a significant difference on the executive path is my very strong work ethic. Hard work is one of our Athabascan Indian values. I work hard because of my passion to give back to my people."

"Also, I was willing to take risks by accepting opportunities that were outside of my comfort zone. The combination of my hard work and my ability to learn quickly and perform helped me to advance."

—Vivian A. Echavarria, FACHE, Vice President,
Professional and Support Services,
Alaska Native Medical Center

"I think one positive quality that contributed to achievement early in my career was taking initiative to volunteer for committees focused on better care for our patients. I had a full plate with work and school but I wanted to be a change agent. Also, my work ethic, perseverance, passion, and drive have helped me to get noticed and advance in my career."

—Eddie Cruz, MBA, FACHE, Vice President of Operations,
Access Community Health Network

Reflection and Action

Look deeper at your own personal qualities and discern how they affect you and your leadership:

- What personal qualities represent who you are as a person?

- Which of these qualities has had the most significant impact on your career journey?

- Which of these qualities has had the most significant impact on your leadership?

- What do you need to do to become more self-aware and mindful about your positive personal qualities?

- What actions do you need to take to develop your positive personal qualities?

CHAPTER 4

The Power of Relationships

Do you think about the types of relationships you have with others and the impact those relationships have on your career journey? For the executives in this book, relationships were powerful contributors to their success. This chapter will discuss the differences that relationships made in their careers.

MEANINGFUL RELATIONSHIPS

Meaningful relationships influenced these executives' advancement to the C-suite. This may sound like a cliché or just common sense, but it is more than that. The connections and close associations that the executives in this study developed and nurtured were essential to their career trajectories. It took more than performance and results for these executives to be recognized, respected, and promoted. Their ability to develop positive relationships was purposeful yet authentic. They were not focused on gaining power; on the contrary, these executives knew that relationships would help them learn and grow and support them in challenging work environments.

The study participants talked about the people who had made a difference in their lives with gratitude and fond remembrances. As they progressed on the executive path, they maintained these connections, and in most cases, their relationships endured. Several types of relationships made a difference: bosses, peers and colleagues, physicians, and developmental relationships, which encompass mentors, coaches, and sponsors. Let's look at each type of relationship and learn about its impact.

BOSSES

Everybody reports to somebody in organizational life. Today's complex team-based health systems comprise direct and indirect reporting relationships. It is important to nurture both. During your career, you will likely report to many different people. The relationships that these executives had with their bosses along their career journeys were critical to their advancement.

What did the good bosses do? They provided leadership and managed performance. In most cases, they provided guidance that the executives required to do their jobs. The bosses who made the most significant impact on the executives' careers were those who acted as sponsors, providing assignments that expanded the participants' leadership and management capabilities. For example, many of the executives talked about receiving stretch assignments for which they had little prior experience and had to learn while they were doing the assignment. These types of experiences facilitated their growth.

In many cases, bosses also acted as mentors, giving both positive and specific negative feedback. In many cases, the study participants did not wait for their bosses to offer feedback—they asked for it, especially negative feedback. They also asked questions and sought guidance on how they could improve their performance. Although positive feedback is important, these executives understood that specific, constructive negative performance feedback would yield the most substantial learning.

The interviews revealed that the executives' relationships with their bosses were authentic, even when they were difficult or challenging. The executives were sincere in their efforts with the intention of wanting to do their best and recognizing that doing so was essential for their career advancement.

On a more personal level, the executives made an effort to get to know their bosses personally and have conversations with them about subjects other than work, such as golfing, boating, running, family, and so on. Rather than focus on their differences, these executives looked for similarities—what they had in common with their bosses. Those commonalities became the focus of their conversations. In this way, they built richer relationships that enabled their bosses to get to know them as people and vice versa.

This approach to developing relationships with bosses aligned with the positive personal qualities that these executives shared (discussed in chapter 3). Qualities such as having a strong work ethic, taking initiative, being willing to take risks, maintaining a positive outlook, being open to learning, and being adaptable facilitated these invaluable relationships. Authenticity and sincerity, along with being values centered, were key.

PEERS AND COLLEAGUES

These executives did not make the mistake of taking their relationships with peers and colleagues for granted. They recognized early in their careers that the people they worked with were important for getting the job done effectively as well as for learning and support. As one said, "Number one, you had to surround yourself with great people." Another affirmed that "surrounding myself with people that I could trust, people that I knew would keep me honest, both inside and outside of the organization" was key. Trust was emphasized again: "I rely on that trust factor and so build trusting relationships with a lot of folks." In today's healthcare organizations, collaboration across multiple boundaries with people you work with directly and indirectly is imperative. These executives understood that fact early on and continued to hone the skill of collaboration to achieve their goals.

For example, one executive said, "The ability to nurture relationships . . . can't be overemphasized." Another recalled that a project "went really well because I had good relationships with the facilities team and plant operations team." Another revealed, "I was very good with relationships." Peers and colleagues acted as sounding boards for sharing ideas and gaining input. In many instances, they became teachers because they had skills and experience that provided valuable learning the executives needed to improve their performance. For example, one person said, "You formed your own little network of people who you could call and say, 'I'm not sure I understand this.'" These peers and colleagues often became mentors who provided emotional and psychological support as well.

At times, peers and colleagues influenced others in the organization by telling people about the good work that these executives were doing. This endorsement enhanced the executives' careers and sometimes led to promotions. As one executive shared, "I have been very fortunate that I have never had to go out and seek a job." He continued, "Relationships built during the previous job led to being recruited for this position." Another concurred: "It was the chain of relationships developed on the job that led to different moves."

An executive summed up the value of peer and colleague relationships this way: "Building positive relationships and navigating relationships" was one of the most significant lessons learned on the executive path. This statement was representative of what all the participants shared in their stories.

PHYSICIANS: CRITICAL PARTNERSHIPS

Physicians are colleagues, too, and everything said so far in this chapter also applies to them. But more than that, physicians play a unique role that is critical to quality, health equity, and organizational performance in hospitals and health systems. Relationships with physicians must be developed and managed in every experience on the executive path. The executives interviewed made a point of describing how working with physicians helped them lead and manage in the organizations on their career journey.

There were a couple of cases, however, in which physicians were not helpful and even were adversarial because they did not like the changes that were being implemented in the hospital. The executives managed these situations by maintaining a purposeful focus on quality patient-centered care. The relationships and respect that the executives had built with other physicians and with colleagues helped them navigate these difficult situations.

A significant lesson learned was that leadership in healthcare delivery organizations depends on working effectively with physicians and viewing them as partners in achieving the hospital's mission and vision. As one executive indicated, "I developed a strong skill set with physicians and was able to work with them." She went on to say that she focused on a win–win approach and was able to gain the medical staff's trust early on. For example, this executive created a physician advisory group that helped guide quality improvement. The physicians acted as confidantes during the change process.

Another said, "I think leadership lessons that come to mind have to do with how I worked with physicians; that is a skill that only comes through experience." A related reflection was, "What I learned . . . was the value of relationships with physicians." A different person reflected on his first chief operating officer position, in which his main function was rebuilding strategic relationships with the medical staff. He worked with the physicians by listening to them, learning about their goals and challenges, and addressing them collaboratively. Similarly, an executive told a story about being a non-clinician with leadership responsibility for a clinical department. She earned respect from physicians by learning as much as possible about the clinical and research aspects of the program so that she could speak the physicians' language and understand issues from their perspective. In doing so, she built a bond with the physicians.

The physician executive in this study believed that being a medical doctor enabled him to have a better understanding of physician needs and challenges. He believed that this understanding enhanced his ability to communicate with other physicians.

An executive captured the collective thinking of all interviewed: "One leadership competency is to be able to collaborate and partner with physicians." Viewing physicians as partners reinforces that they are more than colleagues. Partners share ownership and responsibility for achieving organizational goals and objectives. They have mutual accountability for serving patients, families, and communities. The executives in this study not only understood this, they also acted as role models.

DEVELOPMENTAL RELATIONSHIPS

Developmental relationships had significant meaning for the executives in this study and helped shape their career trajectories. Developmental relationships provide critical support for an individual's career development and organizational experience (Thomas 1990). They are different from other types of relationships in that they help individuals manage challenges associated with their work and with organizational dynamics. Most commonly, the executives interviewed for this study described their experiences with executive coaches, mentors, and sponsors. Each played a different role. As you read their stories, think about your own experiences with developmental relationships.

Executive Coaches

Coaching is a formal and structured collaborative process focused on behavior and performance improvement. This process involves facilitating learning, conducting assessments, and monitoring action plans (Passmore and Fillery-Travis 2011; Reitman and

Benatti 2014). In this study, 7 out of 12 executives worked with a coach when they reached the executive level as an executive vice president, chief operating officer, or CEO. Coaching was often part of an executive development program that included a 360-degree feedback process sponsored by the hospital or health system. In one case, an executive firm was hired to work with the CEO's executive team, and as part of that process, the CEO was required to work with a coach. In another situation, working with an executive coach was part of the CEO's employment contract.

What did the coaches do? They met with their clients to discuss formal 360-degree feedback and guide the learning process associated with it. Executive coaches also observed meetings and provided feedback on the conduct of the meeting with the goal of improving leadership for results. In another instance, a coach was hired for a specific purpose: to improve communication skills.

The executives were fully engaged in the coaching process. They viewed it as an opportunity to enhance self-awareness and to improve their leadership skills. In every case, the executives believed the coaching process helped them achieve their development goals.

Mentors

Mentors play an invaluable role in career advancement and success. This was certainly true for everyone interviewed for this book. Each executive described the impact of mentors on both their personal and their professional development. One of the interviewees described her experience with mentors: "A mentor is a person who will speak truth to you; who will give you advice, solicited and unsolicited; who will help you see blind spots; and who will be honest with you. A mentor is someone who is interested in more than your professional development but [is] also interested in who you are—your personal development."

A broader definition describes a mentor as a person who helps shape the professional identity of the mentee, teaches formal and informal culture in the work environment, provides guidance and psychosocial support, helps navigate organizational politics, assists with engagement in organizational and professional networks, and shares values and skills (Walsh, Borkowski, and Reuben 1999, 270). Both of these definitions reflect the collective experiences of the executives in this study.

Why Mentors

The executives recognized early in their careers that they needed to learn from other professionals who had achieved a high level of success and possessed knowledge that would help them grow. For this reason, they sought out and initiated mentoring relationships. In some cases, the mentors chose them. Indeed, a research study found that "some mentors and sponsors said that they chose people to develop who shared their values and agendas" (Thomas 1993, 190). My research supports this assertion: In most instances, the study participants' values and focus on high achievement were aligned with their mentors.

The executives developed genuine relationships with their mentors focused on learning and psychosocial support. Relationships with colleagues sometimes evolved into mentoring over time as well. And, in many cases, bosses also acted as mentors. Positive relationships with bosses were the foundation of good mentoring. Once they achieved the top executive position, a few individuals described their board chair as a mentor. Other mentors were either internal or external colleagues. Professional networks and associations were good resources for meeting potential mentors.

Working with Mentors

The interviewees identified several lessons about working with mentors. One executive indicated that she would come to her meetings with her mentor with an agenda and follow up on topics discussed in the previous meeting. Another said that he would identify a problem that he had been thinking about, then tell the mentor what he was thinking about it. From there, he would ask the mentor to "poke holes in what he is saying" and listen to the mentor's guidance.

These two examples are representative of how the other executives did not take their mentoring relationships for granted. They understood the importance of purposefully preparing for meetings with mentors. It was essential to identify what they wanted to learn and where they needed guidance. This helped make the meetings more meaningful and results oriented. The mindset of aspiring to learn as much as possible helped make the most of these relationships. The executives also noted that they expressed gratitude for the time and interest their mentors gave them. These were rich relationships that endured over time in most cases.

In essence, working well in mentoring relationships gave these executives the guidance and support they needed to navigate the challenging terrain of the executive path. To make this point, an executive said, "If it weren't for my mentors, I would not be here."

Alternative Perspectives on Mentors

While the majority of interviewees believed that mentors were critical for their career advancement, there was an exception. One of the CEOs indicated that she had not had mentors; rather, she described key people who had supported her journey as "phenomenal partners." Her definition of a phenomenal partner was "someone I could complement or they could complement me from a skill set perspective." She also referred to them as friends. As she talked about these partners and friends, it became clear that they played the role of mentors as traditionally defined. This viewpoint echoes what was said earlier about not underestimating the supportive role that colleagues and peers play in career advancement.

A study on women healthcare CEOs indicated that mentors, although important, are not essential for success (Roemer 2002). However, the women in the study did have supportive relationships. These alternative perspectives give us insights to explore further.

Race and Ethnicity in Mentoring Relationships

Since the interviewees are racially and ethnically diverse professionals, I think it is important to include perspectives on diversity in mentoring. Most of the mentoring relationships explored in this study crossed racial and ethnic lines. There were also same-race and mixed-race/ethnicity mentoring relationships. The two African American female executives interviewed made a point of mentioning that they had had an African American female mentor on their career journeys, although most of their mentors were white women or men. In describing the relationships with African American women, they indicated how much they had learned from them and their ease in having open conversations. One said, "I allowed myself to be a little more vulnerable with her."

In a different case, an Asian American male described his relationship with an African American male who had a significant impact on him as a professional and on his career advancement. His description of this relationship implied that there was a comfort level in developing a close relationship with another male of color. In another case, an Asian American female had a Hispanic/Latino mentor. In describing this relationship, she did not focus on his ethnicity but on the way he acted as a role model who enhanced her own leadership development.

Studies have examined race and mentoring. For example, Morehouse College president and former Harvard Business School professor Dr. David A. Thomas (1990, 1993, 2001) suggests that managers need to be educated on how to mentor and that education should include awareness of differences in cross-race mentoring. According to Thomas (2001), potential obstacles need to be addressed; for example, mentors should be aware of negative stereotypes they may hold about other racial/ethnic groups' ability to succeed. Another obstacle is hesitation to discuss sensitive racial issues that the protégé may be experiencing in an organization. Both mentors and protégés need to embrace racial and ethnic awareness and integrate this understanding into their relationship. At the core of developing an effective cross-race/ethnic mentoring relationship is cultivating mutual trust.

Whether race/ethnicity mattered in the developmental relationships that these executives made was not the focus of my research. However, it is an important factor that deserves further study. What this study demonstrated is that the executives interviewed benefited greatly from the different types of mentoring relationships they experienced.

Sponsors

It takes more than mentors to progress on the executive path. As mentioned in the discussion on bosses, sponsors can play a different role by actually providing opportunities that deepen leadership development and lead to promotions. The role of sponsors is so significant that it is the subject of chapter 5.

SUMMING UP RELATIONSHIPS

The power of relationships lies in your ability and capacity to develop meaningful relationships that enrich your life and career. The capacity to influence others to want to get to know and support you on your journey is for you to develop and broaden. Also, your ability to identify the best people to be in your circle of support is an essential opportunity for you to embrace purposefully. All relationships both formal and informal are potential powerful contributors to your success as a person and leader. Remember, do not take any relationship for granted—even the negative ones. Each one provides a chance for you to learn more about yourself and others. Relationships are the heart of leadership.

KEY LESSONS

- It is important to be sincere in developing relationships. Phonies and manipulators do not get very far.

- Your immediate boss is one of your most essential relationships.
  - It is important to get know your bosses and let them get to know you both professionally and personally.
  - Bosses are often sponsors.

- Peers and colleagues should not be taken for granted: They may become your mentors, sponsors, partners, or friends who help you make progress.

- Physicians are critical partners on the executive path.

- It is helpful to understand the different types of developmental relationships and how to work with them effectively. Mentors are essential. Sponsors are critical for career advancement.

- Recognize and acknowledge conscious and unconscious biases related to race/ethnicity, gender, and other types of diversity. Awareness of biases can help you understand how they affect your relationships. With this awareness, you can work toward developing meaningful relationships built on understanding and appreciation of differences, mutual respect, trust, and seeking common ground.

EXECUTIVE COMMENTARY

"One of my most meaningful relationships was with my preceptor during the administrative residency. It had a positive impact on my career and leadership. I continue to nurture that relationship to this day. As I advanced on the executive path, I saw every relationship as a chance to learn, whether it was a direct supervisor or someone else that was a role model in the organization. Sometimes I would observe how they conducted themselves in meetings or the knowledge and expertise that they brought to a particular project. I was mindful that I was surrounded by people with years of experience and there was wisdom being shared around the table. I saw every interaction as an opportunity for growth."

—Enrique Gallegos, FACHE, CEO, Laredo Medical Center

"Bosses played a significant role in my career. They were both mentors and sponsors that provided encouragement to progress and gave me challenging assignments. One of them introduced me to the value of networking and professional development in ACHE."

—Vivian A. Echavarria, FACHE, Vice President,
Professional and Support Services,
Alaska Native Medical Center

"A lot of people start new jobs and they are very focused on demonstrations of achievement and capabilities and not as much focused on building relationship capital. I think relationship capital is extremely important."

—Dr. Sachin H. Jain, MD, MBA, President and CEO,
CareMore Health

REFERENCES

Passmore, J., and A. Fillery-Travis. 2011. "A Critical Review of Executive Coaching Research: A Decade of Progress and What's to Come." *Coaching: An International Journal of Theory* 4 (2): 70–88.

Reitman, A., and S. Benatti. 2014. "Mentoring Versus Coaching: What's the Difference?" Association for Talent Development. Published August 8. www.td.org/insights/mentoring-versus-coaching-whats-the-difference.

Roemer, L. 2002. "Women CEOs in Health Care: Did They Have Mentors?" *Health Care Management Review* 27 (4): 57–67.

Thomas, D. A. 2001. "The Truth About Mentoring Minorities: Race Matters." *Harvard Business Review* 79 (4): 98–112.

———. 1993. "Racial Dynamics in Cross-Race Developmental Relationships." *Administrative Science Quarterly* 38 (2): 169–94.

———. 1990. "The Impact of Race on Managers' Experiences of Developmental Relationships (Mentoring and Sponsorship):

An Intra-Organizational Study." *Journal of Organizational Behavior* 11 (6): 479–92.

Walsh, A. M., S. C. Borkowski, and E. B. Reuben. 1999. "Mentoring in Health Administration: The Critical Link in Executive Development." *Journal of Healthcare Management* 44 (4): 269–80.

The Essential Role of Sponsorship

IN THE PREVIOUS CHAPTER, we learned about the instrumental role that sponsors play in executive career trajectories. I did not want to leave it there. Sponsorship is a bit more complex than mentorship, and it is harder to attain. What more do we need to learn about sponsorship? Do we need to put more emphasis on sponsorship? Let's take a closer look.

OVER-MENTORED AND UNDER-SPONSORED?

In a 2015 *Harvard Business Review* article titled "Why Men Have More Help Getting to the C-Suite," researchers Solange Charas, Lauren L. Griffeth, and Rubina Malik (2015) explore why women are underrepresented in the executive ranks and suggest that they may be over-mentored and under-sponsored. According to these authors, mentor and sponsor relationships are often viewed through a behavioral lens rather than an economic one—that is, in terms of the economic benefits of being a mentor or a sponsor. The mentor's benefit is intangible, in that he or she feels good about helping another person. However, the sponsor's benefit is tangible: It is measured by the economic expectation that "if you help me, I'll help you"—a traditionally male attribute.

This economic perspective gives us something to consider when exploring the underrepresentation of racial and ethnically diverse professionals in the C-suite and at the executive level in healthcare. Are racially and ethnically diverse professionals being over-mentored and under-sponsored? If so, why? These questions deserve further consideration.

Based on the interviews conducted for this study, it is clear that sponsors significantly influenced the executives' career trajectories. For this reason, I believe we need to put more emphasis on sponsorship and gain a deeper understanding of the relationship and political dynamics associated with it.

THE SPONSOR RELATIONSHIP AND ITS POLITICAL DYNAMICS

If we look at sponsorship from a sociological perspective and consider some original thinking on this topic, we learn why sponsorship is harder to attain than mentorship. We gain insights into the sponsor–protégé relationship and its political dynamics. This perspective gives us viewpoints that are not commonly talked about in healthcare but provide a context for understanding the experiences of the executives in this study.

In a seminal article, Dr. David A. Thomas focuses on the impact of race on managers' experiences with developmental relationships, citing the noted sociologist Dr. Ralph Turner. Thomas (1990, 480) defines sponsorship as the "mechanism by which certain people in an organization are chosen and endorsed for upward movement." This is a critical point, because it indicates that an individual is *selected* for sponsorship. Turner (1960, 856) uses the term "sponsored mobility" to mean that individuals are chosen by established elites based on merit that "cannot be taken by any amount of effort or strategy."

Upward mobility is analogous to entry into a private club that requires new members to be sponsored. The criteria for getting in evaluate whether the candidate has the qualities that the club wants in its fellow members. Turner (1960, 857) expands on this point: "Individuals do not win or seize elite status; mobility is a process of sponsored induction into the elite." One of the women executives interviewed for this study supported this assertation, stating, "You can't ask someone to be your sponsor." This view was implied by other participants in the study.

This meaning of sponsorship suggests that the C-suite is like an elite club, and to get into it, you have to be sponsored. These elites—members of the C-suite and other executives, the majority of whom are white—make decisions about sponsoring emerging leaders based on their performance and whether they think those leaders will be a good fit or have the qualities necessary to become members of the C-suite club. The idea of being a good fit goes beyond performance and results; in practice, it also encompasses such things as personal and social interests and activities. Fitting in may be more challenging for racially and ethnically diverse professionals because they may not have been exposed to the same interests and activities.

Here are a couple of examples: One female executive, whom I call Mary, shared a story about how everyone on the executive team played golf. She felt left out because she could not engage in conversations about golf. What did she do? She learned how to play golf. Another executive, Emily, recalled being invited to go sailing with her boss. She had never been sailing, but she went anyway and found it to be delightful. Emily was willing to try a new experience in an effort to build a better relationship with her boss. That effort paid off, because he became her sponsor. He expanded her responsibilities and provided future opportunities that would accelerate her growth. These are just two examples. In all cases, the leaders in this study understood the importance of fitting in and demonstrating social competence.

Both Turner (1960) and Thomas (1990) give us a deeper understanding of the relationships and political dynamics associated with sponsorship. Mobility to the top must be sponsored, and race/ethnicity and gender can play a role in forming the developmental relationships that make sponsorship possible. For this reason, attaining the C-suite and other senior executive roles can be particularly challenging for racially and ethnically diverse professionals and for women. In addition, these perspectives may explain why some racially and ethnically diverse professionals progress to a certain point on the executive path but do not reach the top. It is important to note that being selected for sponsored mobility starts early in the career journey. Relationships with bosses who often are sponsors are crucial for advancement.

RESEARCH PERSPECTIVES ON SPONSORSHIP

Race/Ethnicity and Sponsorship

Several researchers have offered insights into the challenge of gaining sponsorship into the C-suite and executive level from a race/ethnicity perspective. One group of researchers found that when people of color or women are a minority in organizational settings, a perceived "stereotype threat" may occur (Block et al. 2011). That is, the awareness that an individual may be judged based on negative racial/ethnic or gender stereotypes can result in poorer performance. This research focuses on responses to perceived stereotype threats in the workplace, which can include fending off stereotypes, becoming discouraged by stereotypes, or becoming resilient in the face of stereotypes.

What is the relevance of this research to sponsorship? Think about it—if you hold the negative stereotype that African Americans, Hispanics/Latinos, Asian Americans, or women do not make effective leaders, would you sponsor them for leadership opportunities and positions? Or, if you are a racially/ethnically diverse professional or a woman who believes that no one will sponsor you for senior leadership opportunities because of negatives stereotypes, are you setting yourself up for failure? Negative stereotyping can cut both ways, and it is important to be mindful of your thinking.

Another set of researchers found that in the United States, a key characteristic of leadership is being white and that evaluators perceive white leaders to be the business leader prototype more than racial/ethnic minorities (Rosette, Leonardelli, and Phillips 2008). This phenomenon is referred to as the "white standard." The second part of this study indicated that leader categorization may account for differences in performance evaluations of white and nonwhite individuals, suggesting that whites are evaluated as more effective leaders and as having more leadership potential.

What are the implications of this finding for sponsorship? Bias against racially/ethnically diverse professionals and women may influence who is selected for leadership positions, stretch assignments, advancement opportunities, and access to C-suite leaders because of the white standard. Further research is needed to determine the impact of conscious and unconscious racial/ethnic and gender biases such as the white standard on sponsorship and how these biases are embedded in organizational cultures and systems. With that said, awareness of these biases and how they may impact sponsorship decisions and sponsorship relationships is essential. Awareness can help you navigate structural biases that are deeply rooted in organizational cultures.

When taking into account the impact of negative stereotypes and the white business leader prototype, racial/ethnic minorities and women may have a more difficult time attaining sponsored mobility to the C-suite and executive positions. To simply say that sponsors are essential to advancement on the executive path minimizes the complexity of the challenges that racial/ethnic minorities and women face. However, these challenges are not insurmountable. The executives interviewed in this study did not focus on racial/ethnic or gender biases yet maintained their identities. They focused on mission and performing in service to it. This is the antidote to negativity.

Bear with me for just one more research-based theory that has practical implications for understanding sponsorship dynamics.

Sponsorship as a Social Exchange

Another way to understand sponsorship is to see the relationship as a social exchange. Social exchange theory indicates that human relationships are an exchange of tangibles or intangibles with the intention that some benefit will be derived from the interaction (Homans 1958; Lawler and Thye 1999). If we apply this definition to real-world relationships between sponsors and protégés, it stands to reason that both are engaged in the relationship for mutual benefit. The sponsor is likely looking for some return on investment for giving the person sponsored an opportunity. The return on investment may be partly altruistic, such as helping a colleague succeed, but equally important, the sponsor wants a reward that is tied to the bottom line of the hospital or health system business.

An example is a tangible improvement in quality of care for a specified population. In this case, the sponsor gains the reward of recognition for the business improvement and being an inclusive leader. The protégé gains the reward of recognition for achieving results that will help the health system reach its goals with the potential to enhance career advancement.

The social exchange relationship involves more than just being sponsored for challenging assignments and positions that will enable career mobility. Sponsorship is a valuable win–win business relationship. The executives we have been learning about kept their end of the bargain and produced results that did not disappoint their sponsors. They had a win–win attitude that paid off with opportunities for advancement. This gives you another perspective to consider when you position yourself to be sponsored or to become a sponsor.

SUMMING IT UP

In the real world of healthcare organizations, the complexity of relationship and sponsorship dynamics can be understood from several perspectives: sponsored mobility, conscious and unconscious biases about race/ethnicity and gender, and social exchange relationships. These dynamics are theories in action and realities in organizations. Entry into the C-suite and the executive level requires awareness and management of these sponsorship dynamics if the goal is to attain membership in the elite club. It takes both performance and positive relationships. Based on the perspectives just shared and the practical experiences of the executives in this study, that is easier said than done.

If the elite majority have unspoken criteria for membership into the C-suite, it makes it even more difficult for minorities on the executive path to be admitted. Such unspoken criteria are especially daunting because membership qualifications that are not performance related may not be communicated explicitly; they may only be known among the elites. The elites may not even be conscious that they have unspoken criteria. The adage "birds of a feather flock together"—also known as homophily—has relevance here (McPherson, Smith-Lovin, and Cook 2001). We know that people who have things in common, such as personal interests, social connections, and activities, tend to stick together and may not be open to letting others into the group. It is critical to understand the complexity of sponsorship dynamics and how they may impact racially/ethnically diverse professionals, both men and women.

The executive leaders in this book are good examples of earning sponsorship and successfully developing positive relationships regardless of their race/ethnicity and gender. Here are additional insights from their experiences.

INSIGHTS ON SPONSORS

The majority of the sponsors were white men. Others were white women and racially/ethnically diverse professionals during different phases of their career journeys. In many cases, the sponsors were their bosses. They offered responsibilities that provided the chance for these executives to learn new leadership skills and practical experiences that helped prepare them for next-level-up positions.

In addition, the leaders gained opportunities to manage departments or divisions in which they had limited or no prior experience. An executive whom I call Sarah said, "I was exposed to a lot. It was not that I went to ask for it; they would say, 'You go do it.' and I did it." Another executive made the point that these kind of "you can do it" opportunities came under a mentoring umbrella. In another example, Mary's boss gave her all of the financial departments to lead and manage. She said, "That's how I learned." Both Emily and Paula were given opportunities early in their careers to lead clinical departments, experiences that helped them progress to higher-level responsibilities, which included leading multiple clinical departments.

Similarly, Cheryl was given internal job rotations in every key department of the hospital and gained firsthand experience that helped her understand the whole organization. Alvin, in talking about a new assignment, said, "I had not worked in that magnitude before." He went on to say, "Anytime you have a job that does not scare you, it's probably not much of a job." These were not sink-or-swim situations but rather stretch opportunities that provided valuable real-world experiences that helped these executives progress.

In addition, sponsors made introductions to executives at more senior levels and provided access to leaders that influenced the executives' career mobility. Some sponsors recommended their protégés for positions on task forces, committees, and executive councils that provided practical executive development and exposure. These experiences further enhanced the executives' visibility within the organization, and in some cases regionally and nationally.

The results achieved because of these sponsorship experiences support the findings of research conducted by the Center for Creative Leadership (CCL). Based on its research and practical outcomes of time-tested executive development processes and programs, the CCL developed the "70-20-10 rule." Three types of experiences have a significant effect on executive development: 70 percent on-the-job experiences and challenges, 20 percent developmental relationships, and 10 percent training coursework (CCL 2019). Further, the CCL found that the key sources of leadership learning were bosses, organizational turnarounds, expanded job scope, horizontal moves, and new initiatives. As these findings indicate, what had the most significant impact on leadership learning and career advancement for the executives in this study were real-world job experiences and challenging assignments that their sponsors facilitated.

EARNING AND MAINTAINING SPONSORS

What did the study participants do to earn these sponsorship relationships? In every case, they described their hard work and results. By now, you can see that this is a recurring theme. These executives accepted the challenge of new assignments and responsibilities with a can-do and learning mindset, even in the face of insecurity about doing work that they may not have done before. Along with this attitude, they were willing to take risks. They sought help from mentors and other confidantes to assuage their insecurities about doing work they had never done and new leadership challenges. High performance was the key factor for sponsorship. But performance alone did not earn sponsors—the relationships were crucial. This is not surprising, since we learned earlier how critical relationships are for career advancement.

As the executives described different positions they held on their career journeys, they talked about the quality of their relationships with their sponsors. They were authentic and sincere, characterized by mutual respect and trust earned over time—just like the other relationships described in chapter 4. At the center of their discussions with their sponsors was a clear articulation of expectations, goals, and accomplishments. One study participant suggested that it is important to let people know about your accomplishments and what you want to do. In addition to engaging in meaningful dialogue about work, the executives also shared stories about personal interests they had in common with their sponsors.

The executives often talked about the value of expressing gratitude to sponsors and other people who had helped them advance. They understood that gratitude is important for nurturing and maintaining sponsorship relationships over time. They expressed their gratitude in a variety of ways, but many noted that a simple "thank you" goes a long way toward enriching a relationship.

REMEMBER . . .

Earning sponsors is not only about your performance and results, it is also about who you are as a person and your ability to develop genuine relationships that inspire leaders to want to sponsor you.

Progression on the executive path will not happen without sponsors. Sponsors are crucial for opening doors to the essential experiences that are required for leadership. When those doors are open, be prepared to walk in with the talent and skills you have been developing along the way—a learning mindset, a willingness to take risks, and an openness to making the most of your experiences. That is what the executives in this study did with each opportunity that their sponsors made possible.

KEY LESSONS

- Sponsors are essential to attain the C-suite and executive level.
- Sponsorship is earned.
- Sponsorship is a win–win social exchange relationship.
- It is important to understand the dynamics of "sponsored mobility" and how to manage them.

What do sponsors do?

- Understand and appreciate differences among people from diverse backgrounds
  - Focus on and talk about common interests
- Develop awareness of conscious and unconscious racial/ethnic and gender biases
  - Move awareness to positive action, getting to know people based on who they are and not negative stereotypes
- Provide stretch assignments
- Increase job responsibilities
- Orchestrate job rotations to expand experience and knowledge, skills, and abilities
- Broaden experiences beyond the job, such as appointments to task forces, committees, councils, and high-profile project teams
- Give constructive positive and specific negative feedback and provide encouragement
- Make introductions to senior executives, board members, and community leaders
- Enhance visibility in the organization, in the community, and in professional associations

What do protégés do?

- Understand and appreciate differences among people from diverse backgrounds
  - Focus on and talk about common interests with potential and current sponsors
- Develop awareness of conscious and unconscious racial/ethnic and gender biases

- Move awareness to positive action, getting to know people based on who they are and not negative stereotypes
- Build and nurture positive relationships
- Work hard
- Accelerate performance and achieve results
- Demonstrate initiative by taking on responsibilities beyond the current job scope
- Be open to new experiences
- Seek feedback, especially negative, and use it for continuous improvement
- Embrace a learning mindset
- Communicate and act on career and leadership development goals
- Talk about accomplishments with confidence and humility
- Express gratitude for opportunities

EXECUTIVE COMMENTARY

"You can't ask someone to be your sponsor. You have to have a relationship or connection with them. They have to believe in you . . . being willing to go outside the normal giving advice and extending themselves for you."

—Phyllis Wingate, President, Atrium Health–Carolinas HealthCare System, North East

"Someone saw my potential and elevated me. . . . The passion and conviction to the cause for health equity brings integrity of thought and success in leadership."

—Dr. Ram Raju, MD, MBA, Senior Vice President and
Community Health Investment Officer,
Northwell Health

"Sponsors were primarily my bosses that gave me challenging assignments. However, I took initiative to help even when it was not within my purview of assigned departments or responsibility. I think it is very important that you volunteer for opportunities."

—Enrique Gallegos, FACHE, CEO,
Laredo Medical Center

Reflection and Action

As you reflect on sponsorship,

- What are you doing to earn sponsorship? What are you doing to sponsor others?

- What is contributing to success in your sponsor relationships?

- Where do you see opportunities for improving your sponsor relationships?

- What actions will you take going forward to earn sponsorship and develop win–win relationships?

REFERENCES

Block, C. J., S. M. Koch, B. E. Liberman, T. J. Merriweather, and L. Roberson. 2011. "Contending with Stereotype Threat at Work: A Model of Long-Term Responses." *Counseling Psychologist* 39 (4): 570–600.

Center for Creative Leadership. 2019. "The 70-20-10 Rule for Leadership Development." Accessed May 20. www.ccl.org/articles/leading-effectively-articles/70-20-10-rule/.

Charas, S., L. L. Griffeth, and R. Malik. 2015. "Why Men Have More Help Getting to the C-Suite." *Harvard Business Review*. Published November 16. https://hbr.org/2015/11/why-men-have-more-help-getting-to-the-c-suite.

Homans, G. C. 1958. "Social Behavior as Exchange." *American Journal of Sociology* 63 (6): 597–606.

Lawler, E. J., and S. R. Thye. 1999. "Bringing Emotions into Social Exchange Theory." *Annual Review of Sociology* 25: 217–44.

McPherson, M., L. Smith-Lovin, and J. M. Cook. 2001. "Birds of a Feather: Homophily in Social Networks." *Annual Review of Sociology* 27: 415–44.

Rosette, A. S., G. J. Leonardelli, and K. W. Phillips. 2008. "The White Standard: Racial Bias in Leader Categorization." *Journal of Applied Psychology* 93 (4): 758–77.

Thomas, D. A. 1990. "The Impact of Race on Managers' Experiences of Developmental Relationships (Mentoring and Sponsorship): An Intra-Organizational Study." *Journal of Organizational Behavior* 11 (6): 479–92.

Turner, R. H. 1960. "Sponsored and Contest Mobility and the School System." *American Sociological Review* 25 (6): 855–67.

CHAPTER 6

The Executive Path: A Journey, Not a Ladder

Do you think of your career as a ladder? Do you envision yourself climbing a ladder to reach your career goal? The reality for many of the executives interviewed for this study was that they were *not* continuously promoted to the next rung on a ladder. As you will learn, sometimes a step backward or laterally can be a step in the right direction, giving you the change you need to gain experience and opportunities to demonstrate leadership capabilities. Shifting the metaphor for your career journey can change the way you see yourself learning and progressing.

SHIFTING THE CAREER METAPHOR

The Difference Between a Ladder and a Journey

Metaphors are powerful because the images they call to mind can influence the way we think and behave. The ladder metaphor is frequently used to describe how careers progress. The image of a vertical ladder implies that to advance in your career, you have to move upward, step by step. According to this logic, each step is a move to a higher position or to the top, such as the C-suite. The problem with this imagery is that it does not represent reality. No downward or sideways movements are imagined, and there is no stepping off. But in the real world of careers, there is not always one path going straight up. Some people choose to stop on the path, content with the work they are doing. Others decide to change directions. Thus, a career is more like a journey than a ladder.

What is a journey? A journey is a long process that involves change and challenges, often leading to personal development and growth. This definition describes what the executive path is really like—a journey on a winding path.

The Executive Path as a Journey

The executive path is a lengthy and challenging process in which those who seek it must be prepared to embrace personal change and leadership development. Journeys are unpredictable and sometimes ambiguous, because career choices are not always clear and easy to discern. You can develop a plan for the journey, but you cannot completely control what will happen along the way. The executives interviewed in this study described their experiences as not being a stepwise or linear progression upward. Things happened that they did not predict in their career plans. They talked about moving up, moving back, moving across, and sometimes moving out. Yet they were always learning and growing. They learned how to adapt and embrace the journey.

EMBRACING THE JOURNEY

One executive, Calvin, described his career as "a marathon, not a sprint," suggesting that the journey is a long haul that needs to be traveled in "an impactful way to grow, learn, and reach potential."

The emphasis here is on mindful learning and growth to maximize potential. This was an implicit theme expressed by all the executives in the study. They embraced the nature of the journey. Following are more examples of how they did so.

Lateral Moves

Several executives in the study described lateral positions that afforded the opportunity to take on new responsibilities that broadened and deepened their leadership and management capabilities. For example, they were given opportunities to lead a different department or division. On the surface, these moves might seem to be a step back because of title or scope of responsibility, but really they were steps forward because of the depth and breadth of experience gained.

Not "Stepwising"

Paula reflected on her early career, indicating that she had decided not to keep "stepwising" and took a high-visibility executive staff position working for a system CEO. Later, she purposefully decided to get back on the operations path with the intention of becoming a chief operating officer (COO). Another executive was the CEO of a 126-bed hospital who decided to take a position as a senior vice president and COO of a large two-campus medical center. The title was not CEO, but he had responsibility for a larger organization—a position that broadened his leadership and management capabilities and deepened his experience as an executive.

Mary pointed out that sometimes a position that carries a title that may not seem like a logical step can offer an opportunity to deepen career experience and make a difference. Likewise, Cheryl described her executive path as nontraditional: "I went sideways." In her case, she left a hospital COO position to lead a major capital building project for a new hospital. After completing the project successfully, she returned to the hospital where she had been COO as the new CEO.

Changing Functional Paths

In other cases, individuals changed functional paths. For example, Joseph initially applied his industrial engineering education and experience in two different hospitals and then moved into an administrative leadership role—a COO position for another hospital in a for-profit system. Another case was Bob, who had a law degree and began his work in a non-healthcare setting. He later moved into healthcare administration on the strength of his legal work in the field and the reputation that he had earned.

Five of the executives moved from a clinical leadership path, such as nursing, physical therapy, or medicine, into administrative leadership.

Not-for-Profit and For-Profit

There was only one executive whose career had been mainly in the for-profit sector at the time of the interviews. In four cases, executives had worked for both for-profit and not-for-profit health systems during their careers, transitioning from one to the other. In those cases, the experience they gained in for-profit health systems helped them hone the business discipline that they applied to their work in not-for-profit health systems. It is worth mentioning that some of the for-profit health systems had structured executive development programs that benefited several participants in this study.

Moving Out and On

There were times when it strategically made sense to move out of an organization to obtain new knowledge and skills, navigate different organizational cultures, adapt leadership approaches, or develop new relationships. We will learn more about reasons for leaving a position later in this chapter.

These examples demonstrate that the executive path has twists and turns. Since this research was completed, several study participants are not in CEO positions but remain at the senior executive level. This is another example of the winding path on which movement can go in many different directions.

"All the service lines were given to me at a smaller hospital. I saw it as a demotion but the system CEO wanted me to lead transformational change there. The lesson was, what appeared to be a demotion because of organizational size was really a leadership opportunity that enhanced my career."

—Phyllis Wingate, President, Atrium Health–Carolinas HealthCare System, North East

CAREER GOALS AND STRATEGY ARE NAVIGATORS

A major lesson from the research is that all participants had career goals and a strategy in mind for achieving them. The passion for the mission of healthcare is what energized their goals. That passion proved to be very important when unpredictable events took them off course and they had to reposition themselves without losing sight of their goals.

Career goals and strategy are navigators, but passion steers the course. In every case, the executives had career plans. Some were more formal than others. As we learned earlier, all of the executives began in healthcare, with the exception of one person. In most cases, the executives did not begin with the goal of becoming a

CEO or a top executive in a hospital or health system. This was true even for those who had earned graduate degrees in healthcare or business administration. The goal to become a C-suite leader, and eventually a CEO, emerged later, as these individuals gained experience, enhanced their leadership capabilities, and worked with executive leaders.

One executive, Lois, shared that she had known that she wanted to be an executive early on. That is where she thought she could serve best and have an impact in healthcare. This was a goal that became clearer for all of the executives—that their passion for wanting to help people and make a difference in the health and healthcare of individuals and communities could be realized to a greater extent as a top executive. They wanted breadth and depth. Career strategies and goals were not driven by ego or the desire for power, but rather by their underlying passion and mission.

What do career goals and strategy include? First and foremost, there is clarity about how the goals and strategy can help you to achieve your passion and mission. Goals and strategy are not about titles and positions, but rather what you want to do and where you want to do it in service to your passion and purpose. If it is the executive path, as it was for these study participants, then you need to understand that it is typically a long haul. That understanding and mindset helped these executives to manage the ups and downs inherent in any career. They did not hold unrealistic expectations of how much time it would take to reach the executive level.

Some were on a faster track than others. On average, it took the executives in this study 16 years after graduate school to attain their first CEO or top executive position in a hospital; the shortest time was five years, and the longest time was 30 years. For example, in the five-year case, the study participant had worked for several years as a director in a hospital. At that point, she recognized that a graduate degree would help her advance. After completing a master of healthcare administration degree and a two-year administrative fellowship in a health system, it took another five years for her to attain her first top executive position in a hospital in that system.

The best strategies are steered by clarity of purpose and grounded in values. Values are clear and aligned with the positive personal qualities described in chapter 3. This quote from one of the executives bears repeating: "Whatever you do in your career, you have got to live out your life with your value system in place."

"I will tell you: In my journey I never had a specific 'I want to be this in five years, ten years' or any of that. I want to contribute to achieving the mission. I'm a total team player. I should say I'm not directionless, but I don't set specific career goals other than to continue to grow and learn. I think that might be a little different. Some people do suggest that you have career goals. I think that is OK. I also think it is OK to say you may not know exactly what you want but you want to get better and grow. Do I want to get additional responsibility? Sure. Do I want to make a bigger impact? Absolutely, but that doesn't mean a new title in three years necessarily."

—Maulik Joshi, DrPH, Executive Vice President
of Integrated Delivery and COO,
Anne Arundel Medical Center

REMEMBER . . .

Career growth and advancement is an inside-out job. The person within is the center, grounded when everything else is unpredictable or unstable. Those inner qualities enabled these executives to execute their career strategies. With passion, purpose, vision, and values, it was easier to articulate measurable goals for what they wanted to achieve. In most cases, those goals were tied to action steps for attaining them.

> "You need to take that first step forward to recognize areas of improvement and strength so that you will be able to nourish them like a flower to grow as a healthcare executive."
> —Vivian A. Echavarria, FACHE, Vice President, Professional and Support Services, Alaska Native Medical Center

> "Make sure you know what you really want. It needs to come from some place deeper than surface level. . . . Let people know the path you would like to seek, because when you do that, people will help you."
> —Deborah Addo, CEO, Inova Loudoun Hospital

It is important to understand that these goals and action steps had to be adaptable. We all know that the best career strategies will need to change as life happens and as you change as a person. If your career goals and strategy are fixated on a single path, you may miss opportunities that will enable you to live your passion and purpose. Ultimately, you want to make a difference, and that may happen in ways that you did not originally envision. For example, you may decide that the C-suite is not where you need to be to actualize your passion and achieve your goals. Again, it is not about titles, money, and status—it is about what is in your heart that drives what you want to do. Cheryl, one of the study participants, said, "You should do what you love to do."

The external aspect of career advancement is that people need to know your goals. These executives communicated their career plans and sought guidance from mentors, coaches, sponsors, friends, and significant others. Mary told a story about informing her boss, the COO of the health system, that she wanted to become CEO at one of the hospitals. At that point, she was an assistant vice president of hospital operations. The next move was to become vice president and CEO of one of the system's hospitals. This is just one example of similar stories that made clear how it is imperative to communicate career goals.

DISCERNING CAREER MOVES

Calvin often talked about discernment as he discussed his career moves. Discernment was also implicit in the other executive path stories. As Calvin described it, discernment meant reflecting on where he had been, where he was, and where he wanted to go while keeping in mind the impact that any future move could have on his life, family, and career. Discernment may be defined as the ability to judge well. Good judgment about career moves was integral for these executives' mobility.

Reasons for Changing Positions

The executives' reasons for moving to different positions were typical. Some were recruited to lead significant large-scale transformational changes or turnarounds in other health systems, while others had opportunities for leadership in different and more complex organizations. Others moved to attain a CEO position. In most cases, to attain the CEO position, several career moves were required.

Some executives made moves that were not promotions on the path to CEO. In these cases, the opportunity for growth was more important than a promotion. Executive development primarily occurs while doing the job. These individuals recognized that and embraced these types of experiences.

Another reason that the executives cited for making a move was family. For example, a sick parent needed attention. In a different situation, the position required too much travel and was taking a toll on the executive's family. Some chose positions because their children were in school and their education would be disrupted by a move. In another instance, a husband could not move because of his own work at the time.

Difficult situations presented challenges that triggered some executives to change positions. For instance, a new boss or a change

> "I always tell my students, try something that is uncomfortable, that is outside of your sweet spot, because that's how you are going to learn, grow, and develop both professionally and in terms of your style."
>
> —Maulik Joshi, DrPH, Executive Vice President of Integrated Delivery and COO, Anne Arundel Medical Center

in reporting relationships caused departures. In these cases, the leadership approaches or personalities were so dramatically different from those of the executives that they could not work well together.

In a couple of situations, political mistakes were made, such as not taking an internal promotion that was offered by a top executive. That top executive viewed not accepting the position as a lack of interest and, from that point on, wrote off that individual for future promotions. For another executive, discussing interest in a promotion and sharing a résumé with a senior executive who was superior to the executive's boss caused a problem in the relationship. We will learn more about navigating difficult situations and rebounding from mistakes in chapter 8.

These were the key reasons that study participants changed positions. It was not easy to make these moves. Discernment was essential. What follows are the central factors they had to take into consideration when deciding to make the next move.

Making Decisions About the Next Move

In each case, career moves were not made arbitrarily. A great deal of reflection and discernment was needed. With deep thought about what they had accomplished, mistakes they had made, what they were learning, and where they wanted to go and why, the executives made decisions about their best next move. Career strategy and goals were the framework for decision-making. They were clear about the type of growth they needed to achieve their career goals. As we know, the executive path is risky and unpredictable. They not only survived but thrived by fully embracing opportunities with a positive outlook and perseverance to learn as much as possible. Again, the executives' deeply rooted passion and their purpose to make a difference in healthcare so that they could serve others were their guiding lights. There were other factors that they considered. The following sections discuss several of them.

Assessing Readiness to Make a Move

Are you ready for the next move? Have you accomplished what you came to this organization to do? Do opportunities still exist there that will help you achieve your career goals? These are just a few questions that can help you assess your readiness to make a career move.

Readiness to make a career move is more than answering these questions, however. There is more to it than asking whether you have the right competencies and capabilities to do the job. It is also about your emotional and physical health and stamina. Are you exhausted from the long hours that you are putting into your current job? Do you need to take a break to get some rest and time for reflection? In a couple of cases, the executives in this study took a "gap year" before moving into their next position. During that year, they had time to take stock of themselves and their careers. It also gave them an opportunity to rest, travel, and spend quality time with family and friends. In addition, taking a break can allow time to experiment with other types of positions outside of hospitals and health systems. The risk of this decision, of course, is not being able to get back on the executive path. But in both instances, these individuals were able to do it. The takeaway: Take a wholistic approach to readiness before making the next move.

Geographic Mobility

The willingness to be geographically mobile is a significant factor in career advancement. Nine out of the 12 executives (75 percent) in the study relocated to other states to take positions that would enhance their careers. In several instances, they moved more than two times. The three individuals who did not relocate made that choice because they were continuing to find growth opportunities and making the difference they wanted to make. While relocating is not always required, in most cases it is a necessity for career advancement. As mentioned earlier, in many cases, several moves were made to attain the CEO position.

In addition to career goals, these executives considered the impact of their career choices on their families. A geographic move affects every aspect of your life. Discernment about whether to relocate was a family decision for most.

Looking Beyond the Title

Here is something to remember: Titles can be misleading. In one case, an executive went from being a COO to assistant administrator of a major service line in a hospital double the size. Another executive moved from a position as CEO of a small hospital to become a senior vice president and COO of a large medical center. In a different case, an individual moved within a large health system from CEO to COO to administrator/COO of different medical centers within the system. Later, this person became the top executive of a large hospital, but did not have the CEO title. In health systems, the top executive of a hospital within the system sometimes holds the title of president rather than CEO. In another scenario, a president at the health system level may have multiple hospital presidents and other senior executives reporting to him or her.

The lesson is that judgment about making career moves should not be based solely on title. For the executives interviewed in this study, judgments were made based on their career strategies and goals. And, more specifically, the decisions were made based on what they would be doing in the position and how the job would be aligned with their passion and purpose.

Working with Executive Recruiters

Executive recruiters played a key role in career mobility for many executives in the study. In these cases, they developed good relationships with the recruiters. Recruiters are always looking for top talent, and they track their accomplishments. This is in recruiters' best interests because they are compensated for placing the best people in key positions.

An important observation about the executives who worked with recruiters is they managed their relationships with the recruiters rather than the other way around. This means that before deciding to pursue a position, these executives made sure the position would add value to their careers. They asked a lot of questions to learn about the prospective health system. They recognized that leadership approaches and organizational culture are significant factors that influence whether an individual will be a good fit within an organization. Learning as much as they could before the interviewing and selection process was critical. An additional consideration, mentioned earlier, was the impact on family and lifestyle. Some of the positions that recruiters brought to their attention were not pursued because of one or more of these considerations.

Recruiters are a valuable resource for career advancement, and developing relationships with them can be useful. It is important to learn about positions and consider all the factors involved before deciding to pursue a position. Often, positions sound good on the surface, but upon further investigation, they may not be as they are described or may not be a good fit.

Another consideration for racially and ethnically diverse professionals on the executive path is being viewed as a "diversity candidate." Sometimes recruiters are working for organizations that are specifically seeking candidates who are African American, Hispanic/Latino, or Asian American or who represent other types of diversity. The goal to increase racial/ethnic and gender diversity in healthcare leadership is certainly important. There are a couple perspectives to consider as a diversity candidate. One is that helping to fill the diversity gap in leadership, particularly at the senior level, is an opportunity to make a difference. On the other hand, being viewed as a diversity candidate can have a downside, if that is the primary focus for filling a position. As you are executing your career strategy, you want to be sure that selection is, first and foremost, based on your competence and your capabilities to do the job. The fact that you are "diverse" is a bonus. At times, a few of the executives in this study were diversity candidates. As highly qualified professionals, they continued their track record of success.

NAVIGATING THE JOURNEY

The executive path really is a journey that requires a great deal of reflection and discernment to make the best possible judgments about career moves. Embracing the ups and downs of the executive path and having career goals and strategy steered by passion and purpose helped these executives make wise decisions. These decisions strongly influenced their career mobility. Other factors that maximized their career mobility will be discussed in the next chapter.

KEY LESSONS

- The executive path is a long and challenging journey.
- Movement on the path can go in different directions, guided by your passion, mission, career goals, and values.

- It is important to consciously navigate the executive path journey to maximize growth, learning, and advancement.
- Purposeful discernment and reflection are required to make wise decisions about career moves.
- Personal change and leadership development are intentional.

EXECUTIVE COMMENTARY

"The executive path is no longer a sequential ladder. For me, at least, you always go back to mission. If you align your personal goals with mission, vision, values, and doing the right thing, you are going to find opportunities that align with that. They may be off the ladder in some ways, but I think that is important."

"Another characteristic of the executive path is all about who you work with. It's about finding organizations, people, and teams with whom you share a deep set of values and goals. And that doesn't mean a sequential approach either."

"Healthcare is a team sport. In the past you could individually rise to the top, but now you can only do it by working with others in a collaborative fashion. The characteristic of being a collaborator, bridge builder, and convener; that's how you progress on the path."

"There are several additional lessons for navigating the executive path—learn all the time; always improve; be a great teammate; be passionate about the mission; and be a great executor."

—Maulik Joshi, DrPH, EVP Integrated Delivery and COO,
Anne Arundel Medical Center

"If you are trying to optimize your career by being too deliberate about your career strategies rather than taking a more organic approach, you may miss out on better opportunities. It helps to not be too focused on very specific endpoints and keep an open mind. The most important thing is to align yourself as quickly as you can with your passions."

"People also tend to be a little bit too calculating about needing to go to an organization where everything is working perfectly. I think that oftentimes the greatest opportunity is going to an organization where things are not working perfectly. That's where the greatest mobility sometimes comes because, if things are not going well, there is an opportunity to fix things."

—Dr. Sachin H. Jain, MD, MBA, President and CEO, CareMore Health

---

Reflection and Action

As you reflect on your career journey,

- What are you doing to gain further clarity on your passion and purpose?

- How does embracing the executive path as a journey rather than a ladder change how you manage your career?

- What will you do differently?

- What actions do you need to take to navigate the journey more effectively?

- What do you need to do to enhance your career strategy and goals?

- What are you learning about yourself and your career?

CHAPTER 7

Maximizing Career Mobility

CAREER MOBILITY IS influenced by a confluence of factors and strategies. The previous chapter discussed the dynamic nature of the executive path journey and how it can be managed. This chapter will cover additional strategies to maximize career mobility. As you are reading, think about what you are doing to facilitate your career mobility. Reflect on the strategies presented here and how they pertain to your own career. The following sections present several strategies that the executives interviewed for this book used to maximize their career mobility.

SELF-PRESENTATION

Self-presentation is not a new concept. In fact, social and behavioral scientists have been studying it for years. The sociologist Dr. Erving Goffman (1959) wrote the seminal book on the subject, *The Presentation of Self in Everyday Life.* Self-presentation refers to intentional efforts to manage the impressions of others—that is, a person's public image. We know that others' impressions of a person's ability, attitudes, intentions, and other personal characteristics can have an impact on professional success (Leary and Jongman-Sereno 2017). The executives in this study understood the importance of self-presentation to their careers.

They learned early on that the way they presented themselves could influence perceptions of their capabilities. Several executives shared stories about the importance of appearance. For example, Joseph talked about a division president who looked at everything—nails, shoes, and watch—and about the importance of assimilating. Another executive, Alvin, said, "My presentation [was] important to me in terms of how I presented myself and how I dressed." He went on to say, "I made sure that I didn't . . . give people things to be distracted; tailored suits were not over the edge or flamboyant."

Mary reflected on the early stages of her career journey: "I did not have presence." She continued, "It was an area that I knew I had to work on . . . to be successful, and [I] started thinking, 'I have to look the part.'" Her colleagues at the time were mostly men. These individuals understood that professional appearance was connected to the impressions that others had of them. But they also learned that making a good impression was about more than the way they dressed.

Cultivating a professional demeanor was also essential for these executives. Demeanor is an individual's behavior toward others or outward behavior. It refers to the way individuals carry themselves—the way they stand, professional stance, facial expressions, and gestures. Related to professional demeanor for these executives was etiquette and the way they presented themselves in social settings, such as dinners, receptions, and golf outings. For example, the executives spoke of learning about place settings at black-tie dinner parties and learning how to pair wines. These executives learned through practical experiences and feedback from their bosses, mentors, sponsors, and colleagues. In some cases, they pursued formal training in areas they needed to improve. They understood that professional demeanor often makes the first and lasting impression.

Communication goes hand in hand with professional appearance and demeanor. Time and again, the executives talked about the significance of communicating effectively, both verbally and in writing. These are skills that they continuously improved through-out their executive path journeys. Several worked with mentors or executive coaches to improve their communication skills or engaged in extended education.

Dr. Sylvia Ann Hewlett (2014) refers to self-presentation and all of its attributes as "executive presence" in her book *Executive Presence: The Missing Link Between Merit and Success*. Hewlett describes executive presence as the way an individual acts, speaks, and looks. Consciously being aware of self-presentation and being authentic about it is very important. In all the interviews conducted for this study, no one told any stories about being phony or playacting. These executives were successful because of their authenticity. They learned to develop an executive presence and yet maintained their own identities. The cliché of learning to "play the game" can backfire, because playacting can damage one's integrity and, as a result, diminish respect.

Self-presentation with integrity in a positive and professional manner is imperative for racially/ethnically diverse professionals, women, and other minorities because of negative stereotypes and unconscious biases that can influence people's impressions. The executives in this study acted with positive intent to improve and develop the skills they needed to become the best person and professional they could be.

WORK/LIFE BALANCE

The first article that I wrote for the *Healthcare Forum Journal* was titled "The Balanced CEO: A Transformational Leader and a Capable Manager" (Dixon 1998). It was based on my doctoral dissertation research, for which I interviewed 12 hospital CEOs. One of the lessons I learned from them was the value of work/life balance.

I also learned from my own experience of not doing work/life balance well and the incredible toll that it took on me, both mentally and physically. Unmanaged stress, anxiety, and overwork can cause breakdowns, as it did for me. Dr. Brené Brown (2010) calls breakdowns "spiritual awakenings." Fortunately, in my case, it was an awakening and a tremendous gift of insight into how unbalanced I had become. I was able to recover and move forward on my journey in a much healthier manner.

Balanced professionals are better able to maximize their career mobility than those who are burned out and do not prioritize their self-care. The executive path is demanding—as is any career in healthcare, but the demands are even greater at the executive and C-suite levels. Twelve and 14-hour days are not uncommon. In this environment, work/life balance is difficult to maintain. As several of the executives indicated, there never is a time that you are not connected to the position, but still, it is important to disconnect when possible. One executive, Bob, suggested leaders try not to be glued to the job, but rather to manage it wisely.

In every case, the study participants were mindful of the pitfalls of poor work/life balance. They consciously worked to maintain balance. All but two were married. All but three had children. One executive, Joseph, was divorced and had been a single parent for a period of time. He managed his career and family but indicated that it was "a test of character." Most of the married men had wives who did not work outside the home and supported their husbands' schedules. But these men supported their wives by adjusting their schedules so that they could share meals and spend time with their families.

One of the women revealed that she had taken a position that demanded so much of her time, including weekends, that it took a toll on her marriage. She eventually left that position and saved her marriage. The female executives arranged their schedules so that they could get their children ready for school and eat breakfast or dinner with the family on a regular basis. They also participated in their children's school and sports events. Sarah said, "There are certain things that are very important to me and I am very open about it, spending time with my kids and when I am mom." The single executives made time for family, friends, and outside interests as well.

Here are a few lessons from the executives' reflections on work/life balance:

- Decide what kind of life you want to live.
- It is important to disconnect at times. Set aside time for yourself.
- Know your limits.
- Protect weekends as much as possible.
- Arrange your work schedule to spend time with family and friends.
- Make time for exercise. Take care of your health.

These executives underscored that it is essential to be a whole and balanced person. A balanced person is better able to navigate the executive path journey. Work/life balance is a career mobility strategy because it optimizes your capability and capacity for advancement as a healthy person and leader.

NETWORKING: ANOTHER PERSPECTIVE

Networking is crucial for career advancement. What does networking mean to you? Here, networking refers to the informal process of connecting with people to stay updated, gain and share information, learn what is going on in the organization and in the healthcare field, and find out about jobs. Importantly, it is a process of building meaningful relationships for mutual benefit—networking must be reciprocal. This was certainly the case for the individuals interviewed for this study. Both internal and external networking played a role in their career trajectories.

All of the executives were involved in professional associations. The American College of Healthcare Executives (ACHE) and the

National Association of Health Services Executives (NAHSE) were mentioned by several participants as organizations that provide excellent networking opportunities. Those who did not belong to these associations participated in other professional networks and affiliations. Taking on a leadership role in a professional association can enhance visibility and provide another avenue for career development. It is a way to broaden contacts and learn about other organizations. Long-term meaningful relationships are frequently products of engagement in professional associations.

In this age of social media, with LinkedIn, Facebook, Instagram, and Twitter, it is interesting that none of the interviewees cited these platforms as significant for their career trajectories. While having 500 contacts on LinkedIn, for example, might broaden your connections, it may not yield the depth of relationships needed for colleagues to really get to know you beyond your résumé. However, executive recruiters do use LinkedIn and other online career systems to identify potential candidates, so it is important use social media platforms wisely. The study participants spent a great deal of time describing much deeper relationships than can be achieved online. What made the difference in getting a sponsor, a recommendation, or a reference was getting to know the person they were connecting with.

Another point about internal networking: As we learned in chapter 4 on relationships, colleagues within your organization can be valuable sources of information, collaboration, and support. They can help you not only to do your job but also to learn what is going on beyond your department, division, hospital, or health system boundaries. To this point, the executives talked frequently about how they formed internal networks that became valuable partnerships for accomplishing their goals. For example, after being selected for a CEO position, one executive found out that colleagues from her previous organization had been contacted informally to learn about her work and reputation. She had built a successful track record there through high achievement and positive relationships with her colleagues. Using informal networks for reference checking is common. Performance and relationship capital were instrumental in securing the CEO position for this executive. This is just one example of many that were shared by the interviewees—underscoring that it is important to network within your organization and within the broader system or field.

Purposeful internal and external networking are invaluable. Building networks of sincere, mutually beneficial professional relationships can have an exponential effect on career mobility.

> "I think that having a support group of peer colleagues to network within organizations such as NAHSE and ACHE is helpful. We are a sounding board for each other. Your peer group helps keep you grounded and provides encouragement."
>
> —Rick L. Stevens, FACHE President, Christian Hospital

Insights About Race and Ethnicity in Networking

Since the executives in this study are racially and ethnically diverse, I want to share a few insights about race and ethnicity in professional networking. These insights are not an outcome of this research study, but they are relevant for you to think about and explore. Some research has been conducted on the topic of race, career results, and networking interactions. However, there is an opportunity for more to be conducted specifically in healthcare.

Here is an important finding that has relevance today: Racially and ethnically diverse professionals will have the greatest opportunity for advancement when they develop a mix of same-race and cross-race networking relationships (Ibarra 1995; Thomas 1993). Same-race relationships provide psychosocial support, strategies for managing racial barriers, sources of information, and career development role modeling. Cross-race networking can be helpful for professionals working in a majority white context and may offer psychosocial support and career development role modeling. In addition, cross-race networking may be more instrumental in offering career advancement opportunities, particularly when racially and ethnically diverse professionals are a minority. In this context, cross-race networking may provide information that is not available in same-race circles. The takeaway is that racially and ethnically diverse professionals working in predominantly white organizational contexts will likely benefit from both same-race and cross-race networking relationships to maximize their chances for advancement.

On a related note, a recent study that focused on African Americans found that they sometimes find it difficult to build deeper relationships across racial boundaries, particularly in work-related social situations (Phillips, Dumas, and Rothbard 2018). African Americans may not be as comfortable opening up and sharing personal information about themselves in cross-race informal social events. The researchers suggest that this applies to anyone who is a minority in an organization. The reason is homophily—that is, people are more comfortable forming close relationships with others with whom they share common interests and backgrounds.

If you want to progress on the executive path, you will need to be intentional about learning about and from people who are different from you. Rather than focusing on your differences, focus on what you have in common with others. This was mentioned many times by the study participants and by several of the commentators. Opening up and letting people get to know you will help you build richer relationships. People are more likely to want to sponsor and mentor racial and ethnic minorities when they know them well and feel comfortable working with them.

DON'T BURN BRIDGES

I cannot say enough about the importance of not burning bridges. By this I mean ending a relationship in a negative way so that the connection is broken and no longer provides a bridge to the future.

Unfortunately, bad memories tend to last longer than good ones. A broken relationship with a boss can be tragic. A breach of trust with a colleague, whether within an organization or in external networking, can damage your reputation. In life and work, not all relationships will be positive, but how they are managed can either boost or break a career.

For instance, one executive described a situation in which a relationship with the CEO had changed for the worse because of differences in their thinking about the organizational strategic priorities and values of the health system. This executive decided to leave, although the CEO wanted this person to stay. The departure was managed in a constructive manner with effective communication and appropriate time for the transition. Later, at the suggestion of a colleague, this executive decided that it was important to mend the relationship with this CEO. A meeting was set up, and they were able to reestablish their relationship in a positive manner. As it turned out, the hiring CEO for the executive's next career move served on a board with that CEO. They had an informal conversation about this individual that was positive, helping the hiring CEO make the final decision.

The executives in this study told stories about previous bosses and colleagues who not only gave formal references but also made informal comments about the executives as they progressed on their journeys. Informal networks can be powerful sources of information. Here is another example that highlights this point: In this case, the person achieved the first CEO position and later was told how much previous colleagues had contributed to this achievement. Apparently, these colleagues, including many physicians, knew people at the new organization and during the interviewing process shared information informally about this individual. It was good information about accomplishments, the person, and the respect that had been earned.

The takeaway: Don't burn bridges on your career journey! You never know who knows who and may be talking about you.

STEP UP TO DO MORE

In every case, the executives interviewed stepped up to do more than their positions required. This is a theme that runs throughout this book, but it bears repeating because of the impact on career mobility. Beginning early in their careers, the executives initiated opportunities to learn and do more than their job descriptions required. Sometimes that meant volunteering to work on a project with colleagues in a different department, division, or hospital as a way of learning more about a function or area. Sometimes the executives had no prior experience doing what the extra assignment, team project, or committee needed. But they were willing to take a risk, and they knew that by participating in new assignments, they would grow professionally. Importantly, this was not done at the expense of work/life balance, but it was not easy.

In doing so, the executives gained leadership development experience in the most effective way—learning by doing the job. They also gained recognition and respect for being go-getters who wanted to make a contribution to the organization. They demonstrated performance excellence, resulting in promotions down the road.

SAY YES TO OPPORTUNITY

Saying yes to opportunity was another common theme on the subject of career mobility. The executives were willing to take on responsibilities and challenges to enhance their leadership skills. An example is Ralph, who talked about a career move from the clinical leadership path. He revealed that in taking on administrative responsibility, which he had never done before, he was given incredible access to top leaders in the hospital. Eventually, the experience led to his first CEO position.

Other executives spoke of being asked to take over a department and turn it around. The executives took on these kinds of opportunities even when they had limited knowledge of the new department. They achieved outstanding results and gained a great deal of leadership capital. In one case, an executive was given the opportunity to lead a hospital transition. The response was, "Of course, I was going to try it; I figured that I would just figure it out."

The willingness to say yes to opportunity paid big dividends in depth of experience, knowledge, skills, and abilities. And, importantly, these executives were recognized for their leadership.

LEARNING MINDSET

By now you understand that learning is essential to your career trajectory. Inquisitiveness and curiosity are key characteristics of the learning mindset. A mindset is an approach to thinking—a way of seeing things that, in some ways, can lead to a way of being. In line with Dr. Carol Dweck's (2012) "growth mindset," these executives turned every experience into an opportunity to develop their leadership and management competencies. Learning mindfully meant that these individuals consciously and intentionally sought to learn as much as they could throughout their journeys. They were purposeful about it. This was the case even in the most difficult and challenging situations.

Here are several of the executives' comments on the learning mindset:

- "I had an opportunity . . . to build my toolkit."
- "Learn, don't panic" (referring to challenging situations and new experiences).
- "I took full advantage of it."
- "I learned a lot from him [the boss] just by observing."
- "I was always willing to learn new things."
- "I learned about leadership that I did not want to emulate."

- "[My boss] created an environment for me as a new executive that it was OK to make mistakes. He wanted me to ask the questions I didn't know. That's why I was able to grow there so quickly—because I would ask the questions that other people weren't asking."

It is clear that learning mindfully facilitated advancement in every case.

The career mobility strategies described in this chapter are not inclusive of all that must be done to progress on the executive path. They do represent strategies that made a significant difference for the executives in this book.

KEY LESSONS

- Self-presentation and professional demeanor are intentional efforts to manage what people see and hear in a positive manner.

- A whole, healthy, and balanced person can better maximize career mobility.

- Racial and ethnic minorities will likely have greater career advancement opportunities by engaging in same-race and cross-race networking relationships.

- Racial and ethnic minorities may need to work on letting people get to know them in work-related social settings. People are more likely to want to mentor or sponsor those they know well.

- It is important not to burn bridges—the journey can go both ways.

- Strive for excellence in meeting the expectations of your position and look for ways to do more. But do not lose your balance.

- Saying yes to opportunities will enable you to gain new leadership skills and expand your knowledge and abilities, giving you a chance to shine.

- Mindful learning takes place by consciously and intentionally making every experience a learning opportunity.

- Being centered in positive values and personal qualities helps guide and sustain balance during challenging times.

EXECUTIVE COMMENTARY

"I sought out positions that were good for me based on my career goals. It is important to know what you want to attain. Also, it is knowing that you have to make that decision and not rely on others to push you in that direction. This requires self-motivation and initiative. You are the architect of your success."

—Enrique Gallegos, FACHE, CEO Laredo
Medical Center

"We need as individuals to maintain our own health. There is an utmost need for work/life balance. You have to be able to disengage from your work so that you have the balance to be with family."

—Vivian A. Echavarria, FACHE, Vice President,
Professional and Support Services,
Alaska Native Medical Center

"Sometimes I think we get so busy in the doing that we don't pay attention to the learning."

—Deborah Addo, CEO, Inova Loudoun Hospital

"It is important to be intentional about where you work. I believe there are cultures that are much more conducive to success for women and people of color."

"Work in organizations that support work/life balance. I don't judge my success only on my work. My family is my greater success."

"Experience in both staff and line roles, in many divisions of healthcare, has contributed to my success."

—Denise Brooks-Williams, Senior Vice President and CEO, North Market, Henry Ford Health System

"My heart is in community health; that's my passion. Patients shouldn't have to leave their community to access great healthcare. It's about how do we provide better outcomes for patients, especially those most vulnerable. This passion has facilitated my career trajectory, beginning as a hospital orderly, advancing to become a receptionist in a community health center, and through a series of promotions eventually becoming vice president."

"Another essential point about career mobility is that you need to let your boss, boss's boss, and mentors know what you aspire to be. Also, it is important to be present at meetings and make contributions, recognizing that you do have something to offer to the group."

—Eddie Cruz, MBA, FACHE, Vice President of Operations, Access Community Health Network

"There were two key components that contributed to my career success, particularly early career. One was working with a company large enough where I could be promoted within. Being a woman and African American is not easy, especially if you are not in an organization where they are getting to know you. Another critical component was having two significant sponsors during my career."

"Competence will not necessarily get you there. You have to take some risks, actively attract sponsors, and work for organizations where you will fit and where they will be open to you."

—Phyllis Wingate, President, Atrium Health–Carolinas
HealthCare System, North East

Reflection and Action

As you reflect on your career mobility,

- Which approaches discussed here are working well for you?

- What approaches are not working well?

- What actions will you take to maximize your mobility?

- Are there any approaches not discussed here that are working well for you? Share them with your colleagues and friends.

REFERENCES

Brown, B. 2010. *The Gifts of Imperfection: Let Go of Who You Think You're Supposed to Be and Embrace Who You Are*. Center City, MN: Hazelden.

Dixon, D. 1998. "The Balanced CEO: A Transformational Leader and a Capable Manager." *Healthcare Forum Journal* 41 (2): 26–29.

Dweck, C. 2012. "Mindsets and Human Nature: Promoting Change in the Middle East, the Schoolyard, the Racial Divide, and Willpower." *American Psychologist* 67 (8): 614–22.

Goffman E. 1959. *The Presentation of Self in Everyday Life*. Garden City, NY: Doubleday.

Hewlett, S. A. 2014. *Executive Presence: The Missing Link Between Merit and Success*. New York: HarperCollins.

Ibarra, H. 1995. "Race, Opportunity, and Diversity of Social Circles in Managerial Networks." *Academy of Management Journal* 38 (3): 673–703.

Leary, M. R., and K. P. Jongman-Sereno. 2017. "Self-Presentation: Signaling Personal and Social Characteristics." In *Social Signal Processing*, edited by J. K. Burgoon, N. Magnenat-Thalmann, M. Pantic, and A. Vinciarelli, 69–78. Cambridge, UK: Cambridge University Press.

Phillips, K. W., T. L. Dumas, and N. P. Rothbard. 2018. "Diversity and Authenticity." *Harvard Business Review*, March/April, 132–36.

Thomas, D. A. 1993. "The Dynamics of Managing Racial Diversity in Developmental Relationships." *Administrative Science Quarterly* 38 (2): 169–94.

CHAPTER 8

When the Going Gets Tough

THE GOING CAN get tough on the executive path. No matter where you are on the journey, you will encounter difficult situations and difficult people you will need to work with. That can be particularly challenging if the difficult person is your boss. Sometimes difficult situations are created by the boss, or they may be the result of organizational politics or culture. And, of course, you will experience mistakes and setbacks that make the journey tough.

As you will learn in this chapter, difficult experiences are the greatest teachers. Anyone who wants to rise to the executive level must learn to manage difficult people and situations. How you manage these challenging relationships and circumstances can make or break your career. In this chapter, you will learn how the executives in this study smoothed out the rough patches on their journeys. This chapter will cover working with challenging bosses, managing difficult situations, and handling mistakes and setbacks. The following sections describe scenarios based on the stories shared in the interviews.

As you read this chapter, think about the tough times that you have experienced. How did you manage them? How can you use the insights gained from this chapter to help you deal with rough patches going forward?

WORKING WITH CHALLENGING BOSSES

As we discussed in chapter 4, relationships with bosses are critical. On the executive path, you will have many bosses. This is particularly true in today's complex, team-based healthcare organizations. You may have more than one boss at a time. Odds are, not all of them will be easy to work with. Some may have difficult personalities or exhibit negative behaviors. The following sections provide several examples of challenging bosses and how the executives interviewed in this study managed the relationships.

Failure to Promote

One executive, Emily, had accomplished significant results in a senior middle management position, yet she was still not being promoted to vice president. She asked her boss, a senior vice president, what it would take to be promoted. He suggested that she ask the hospital CEO. In a conversation with the CEO, Emily was told that she needed more exposure. This response was shared with her immediate boss, who told her that was not the whole story. The boss went on to say that the top executive group believed that there was a trust issue with her. This feedback was surprising in light of her high performance and strong relationships.

As it turned out, a senior executive in the organization had been perpetuating a lie about Emily's honesty. She eventually discovered that this belief was based on a presentation she had given, during which the senior executive had gotten the impression that she was not taking ownership for negative financial results and blaming the issue on somebody else. What the senior vice president described was not accurate based on Emily's recollection of her presentation.

At that point, Emily had to decide whether to stay or leave. She made the decision to stay and to continue to achieve stellar results and demonstrate integrity. The solid reputation she had earned over time outlived the negative accusation. The senior executive who had made the accusation eventually left the hospital. Emily was offered a promotion, but it was too late, and eventually she left the organization.

Key points: Be persistent in gaining clarity about performance feedback and any misinformation about work or character. Work hard to achieve stellar performance results and maintain positive relationships. Stick with it, but know when it is a no-win situation.

Negative Communication Approach

Two study participants had bosses who yelled at them and used a nasty tone of voice when speaking. In both cases, the individuals stayed in their positions but maintained their self-respect by giving their bosses constructive feedback about their communication approach.

Key points: Use "I" messaging to describe how a person's behavior affects you. Set clear expectations for how you expect to be treated as a professional and as a colleague.

Personality Clash

Alvin described his relationship with one of his bosses as being like "night and day." The boss was a mechanical, data-driven person. After some difficulty in the relationship, Alvin began giving his boss detailed reports and timelines. "I needed to function for a period of time the way he functioned. . . . In order for me to change things, I had to meet him on his terms."

Key points: Get to know your boss and gain clarity on his or her expectations for delivering results. Understand how the boss best receives information. Remember, people have different learning and personality styles. Alvin advised, "Learn how to manage your manager."

Dishonesty

Bob had a former boss who told people that he had been fired, when in fact he had resigned. The leaders in Bob's new organization knew that he had not been fired. However, it was like a dark cloud that the previous boss had put into the community. Even though the people who mattered knew the truth, it was still difficult for Bob to deal with the lie.

Key points: Bob concentrated on performance and results in his new position. As he indicated, he had a choice to make in this situation: "either be angry and let it destroy me, or try to understand the human being and what they did and forgive them." He chose to forgive his former boss and focused on what mattered most—providing quality healthcare to the community.

Limiting Assignment

In another situation, an executive was given an assignment by a new boss to work with a program for low-income Hispanics/Latinos. He believed he was assigned the project because he was Hispanic/Latino, and he felt pigeonholed. There were other assignments that would have helped him learn more about hospital operations, which is what he wanted to do at the time. He revealed that for a while, he pouted about the assignment. But once he decided to focus on using his skills and creativity to improve healthcare services for this population, he was able to transform the program.

Key points: The lesson from this experience: "Don't pout too long. . . . There is a silver lining in everything."

Unsupportive Boss

Joseph talked about an unsupportive CEO boss. At the time, Joseph held the chief operating officer (COO) position. Speaking about how he managed working with his boss, Joseph said, "Learn what you can. My attitude was [that] unless you are doing something unethical or illegal, you are the captain of the ship and I'm your COO. My job is to make it as successful as possible. It is a learning opportunity for me, too. One day I will be captain and I will have the right to choose. You can't pick your leaders. They pick you. So, when given the recognition that I can't pick my leader at the moment, I could leave my job, but I can't be changing jobs every time I don't like somebody. What is the best I can learn from this leader as a takeaway to build my toolkit as I move on?"

Key points: When you encounter an unsupportive boss, strengthen your support network. Learn as much as you can and make the best of the relationship.

Competitive Staff Relationships

In another case, the CEO's style was to facilitate competition among the staff. In effect, he pitted staff against each other. Sarah reported to him and shared her approach to managing this relationship. "I found myself . . . disassociating . . . from what I was feeling about the CEO and the things he was doing to me. The rest of it was all focused on the hospital—running the facility and relationships with the physicians, CNO, and staff." Sarah focused on providing quality patient care. She said, "We all are going to focus out here and then deal with the CEO." The CEO often was not there, and the staff had the freedom to run the hospital.

Key points: Focus on doing what is right for the hospital and patients. Recognize the boss's dysfunctional behavior and do not fall into negative traps. Maintain a positive outlook.

Jealousy

In another case, the CEO was jealous of Cheryl's group's teamwork and closeness. Cheryl and her direct reports met weekly and engaged in robust conversation. Together, they solved problems and learned from each other. The CEO sometimes did things to break up the group. The boss was nice to Cheryl to her face but then would do things behind her back. For example, while Cheryl was on vacation, the CEO made a lot of organizational changes. However, the boss did not undermine her on a daily basis and gave her leadership opportunities. Cheryl indicated that she managed all of this by focusing on the work and not on the distractions. She was successful.

Key points: Focus on the positive aspects of the relationship rather than the negative. Be aware of what the boss is doing and understand his or her motives. Focus on the work and achieving collective goals.

Key Themes for Working with Difficult Bosses

These examples highlight the different types of challenging bosses. Everyone will likely have at least one bad boss on their career journey. The participants in this study were no different, and some had more than one. They learned how to manage their difficult bosses, recognizing that leaving the organization was not the easy answer.

The key theme in each example is that the executives focused on doing their best work and what was right for the hospital. Eventually, either the boss left or the executive chose to pursue a better opportunity. Another valuable point is that these executives learned a great deal by staying as long as they could make difference without causing harm to themselves.

MANAGING DIFFICULT SITUATIONS

Working with a challenging boss is difficult. But a difficult situation is bigger than one person. It may involve multiple people, the whole organization, or some segment of it. The executives in this study told many stories about managing difficult situations. In fact, these tough circumstances are the norm on any career journey. Figuring out how to navigate them is essential for career advancement. Here are a few examples of how these executives did so.

The "Only" Minority

One executive spoke of being the only African American male in management. The administrator viewed him as aggressive, and a seasoned physician with whom he had to work closely was not open-minded. This was the first time the executive found himself in a "pretty ugly situation." It was an eye-opener, he explained, because he had to find a way to surround himself with people he could trust. It was a lesson in realizing that some people would set him up, if it was in their best interest to do so. He was accused of doing some things that were later proven to be untrue.

Eventually, the executive worked through the situation and maintained his self-respect. He said, "I recognized you can't deny performance. . . . I had to make sure, in light of those things, [that] I had to remain productive and not provide ammunition for somebody to bring me down." A lesson he learned was to "focus more on the business at hand and not get immersed in the socialness of it. . . . I realized that sometimes I had to be less of me and more of what the situation required."

Key points: Performance and achieving stellar results are essential. Act with integrity. Develop relationships with people you can trust and seek feedback from them. Adapt your behavior as the situation requires without losing your self-respect and self-esteem. Learn as much as possible about yourself and leadership in a difficult situation.

Physician Leader Performance Problem

In another case, an executive needed to address some quality concerns with a physician leader in the hospital. Other physicians were aware of these concerns but did not want to get involved. She decided to stop a surgical procedure that had significant quality concerns. This action was taken after informing the CEO, who was already aware of the problem. After the physician leader was informed of the decision, he planned to seek the executive's resignation at an upcoming medical executive committee meeting. He came to this executive before the meeting and threatened to have her fired if she did not back down.

The executive had a difficult conversation with him in which she said, "I'm going to do what is right and sometimes that's not always popular." She explained that an important lesson was to stay calm and logical and not take the situation personally. However, the physician made it personal, telling her, "The problem with you is your race and gender." She responded, "I'm sorry that is how you think; I'm going to have to do what is in the best interest of patient care."

The Medical Executive Committee met the following week. In preparation for this tough meeting, she made sure her facts were in order. She also prepared emotionally so that she would remain calm in the face of attack. The meeting went into executive session, and the physician tried to persuade the committee to give a vote of no confidence in the executive. In the end, a majority of physicians voted in her favor. She reflected on this experience and the lessons she had learned from it: "I stuck to my values, which is why I was there—to take care of patients."

Key points: Do what is right for the organization and for patient care. Remain calm under pressure, centered, and grounded in positive values.

First-Time CEO: Transformational Change

In several cases, executives in their first CEO or top executive position faced difficult situations related to organizational change. In one case, the previous top executive had been fired, and the board chair had expanded the boundaries of that role to include operations. The allegiances of the executive team were confounded by the board chair's behavior and their role in bringing about the previous leader's demise. As a result of the disarray at the top, the entire hospital had to be turned around.

In another situation, a health system had had multiple CEOs, resulting in a lack of leadership stability and teamwork. The system was financially unstable and in jeopardy of losing its accreditation. Relationships with unions were fractured. To say to the least, this was a troubled organization that needed to be transformed.

In two different cases, hospitals struggled with mediocre quality and financial challenges. The senior leadership groups were not functioning as teams. Physicians were not performing as expected and demonstrated poor quality outcomes. A couple of clinical programs had to be shut down. In both situations, the new top executive had to lead transformational change.

Key Themes for Managing Difficult Situations

Several key themes for managing difficult situations emerge from these examples:

- Focus on the healthcare mission and your role in helping to achieve it.

- Understand and navigate organizational culture change and political dynamics.
- Build positive relationships with physicians while holding them accountable for quality outcomes.
- Develop effective teams and teamwork with all stakeholders.
- Manage financial challenges ethically.
- Surround yourself with people whom you can trust and who can support you.
- Learn as much as you can about yourself and leadership.
- Be your best self and do your best work.

Navigating tough situations involves more than the foregoing examples might suggest. But the lessons from these executives help us learn what it takes to thrive during difficult times. Their ability to succeed in these circumstances helped them to gain recognition for their leadership capabilities and facilitated their career advancement.

REBOUNDING FROM MISTAKES AND CAREER SETBACKS

Everyone is bound to make mistakes and have setbacks on the executive path. The following examples describe how the executives in this study rebounded from their mistakes and setbacks.

Taking a Wrong Turn

Paula left a senior operations position to take a highly visible senior executive staff position reporting to the new CEO of a large health system. It was an internal move with the goal of fast-tracking to COO. She expected to use this position to learn about all of the system hospitals and career opportunities. After about a year, a hospital COO position became available. However, Paula was not selected because the hospital CEO wanted to bring in his own COO. She was disappointed, and her choice was viewed as a mistake at the time because the strategy for attaining the COO position did not work out. However, it was a tremendous learning experience.

Paula's reflection on this experience was that you cannot be angry; rather, you have to stay the course and keep doing good work. The next step was a decisive move back to the operations track at the vice president level.

Key points: Taking risks and making mistakes provide valuable lessons. To rebound from mistakes, it is necessary to learn mindfully and make course corrections.

"Jumping into the Deep End Without a Life Preserver"

In another case, the health system CEO asked Mary, the top executive of one of the hospitals, to turn around a troubled hospital within the system. He painted a very dim picture of the hospital. Two major service lines were at risk because the chief medical directors were distracted trying to forge alliances with external entities. The financials were not meeting expectations. Mary admitted that the opportunity sounded like a good challenge, and if everything worked out, it would be a career booster. In the past, she had moved every year and a half, and it was about that time, so she took the opportunity. In hindsight, however, taking the position turned out to be one of Mary's biggest mistakes: "I jumped into the deep end and there was no life preserver."

Approximately a year and a half into the position, Mary had achieved significant results that were aligned with the system CEO's expectations. The physician leaders were back on board. The service lines that had once been at risk were making money. But then there was a major shift in the system CEO's performance expectations for that hospital, which were the exact opposite of the original plans. It would mean a shift in mission and values. Following through on the new plan would have caused Mary to lose credibility in the organization after all she had done to turn it around. This was a significant setback. Mary's mentors helped her make the difficult decision to leave the organization.

With a great deal of discernment and support from mentors and family, Mary decided to take a gap year before accepting a new position. The gap year gave her a chance to relax, travel, spend time with her children, volunteer, and, importantly, reflect on her life and career. The story has a happy ending: Mary got back on track after two moves and became the COO of a medical center with additional health system responsibilities.

Key points: Acknowledge mistakes and take time to reflect on how best to recover. Rely on your positive values and qualities to help you discern the situation. Seek support from mentors, trusted advisers, family, and friends. A gap year has risks, but it can be an invaluable way to rebound from a mistake and move forward.

A Political Mistake

At one point on his career path, Tom was a vice president at a medical center that was part of a larger health system. His responsibilities included administrative leadership for multiple functions within the entity. A new health system CEO came on board and offered Tom a promotion to work at the system level as a senior vice president. This role encompassed nonoperational responsibilities such as construction and special projects. The system CEO advised Tom to think about it and let him know his decision.

Tom went to his direct boss to share this information and found out that he already knew about the offer. This was somewhat surprising, since the previous year had been challenging. Tom had a steeper learning curve than in previous roles because of the increased responsibility managing multiple departments and the need to delegate responsibility, relying more on the team. Tom's recent performance feedback indicated that he needed to meet deadlines in a timelier manner as a result of this transition. He had made improvements in his ability to manage broader responsibilities. Tom's goal was to continue growing in operations. Working with a coach proved to be helpful during this time. Tom decided not to take the promotion. Once the decision was made, Tom's immediate boss was informed and then the system CEO.

As it turned out, Tom's decision was a political mistake. From that point on, his interactions with the system CEO changed for the worse, and his opportunities for promotion stalled. He believed that no matter what achievements he attained, they would no longer matter in this organization. It was the end of a long relationship and many accomplishments in that organization. Tom's decision to leave was not easy and took a great deal of discernment. Several months later, Tom took a position as a vice president with another health system. He described this as a tremendous learning experience.

Key points: New leadership often brings changes such as reorganizations, shifts in leadership positions, and different strategies for achieving organizational goals. It is important to understand the political dynamics of new leadership. This is a good time to think about career strategy and goals. Be aware of the consequences of not accepting internal offers. Seek support from trusted advisers such as mentors, coaches, and colleagues. Be sure to weigh all the options, both internal and external. Know when it is time to leave an organization. Exit in a positive manner, remembering not to burn any bridges.

Additional Mistakes and Setbacks

In addition to these examples, the executives described other types of mistakes and setbacks. Here are a few cases:

- One executive was working with a very difficult boss and talked about the situation with colleagues. A colleague or two let the boss know what was being said about him. The relationship was eventually rebuilt, but it was a long and difficult process. **Key points:** Think before you speak. Share confidential information only with trusted colleagues.

- Another executive had had failures on the executive journey, particularly early on. All of them were under an umbrella of high performance and results. They included poor hiring selections, starting programs that failed, and being too direct and aggressive with the boss. She viewed each failure as a learning opportunity and continued to grow. For this reason, her mistakes and failures were facilitators for advancement—that is, for "failing forward." **Key points:** Mistakes and failures are the biggest teachers. Learn and grow from them.

- In another case, an executive expected everybody to come to work with the same drive and intensity that he brought to the position. **Key points:** Everybody has different approaches to work based on their background, experience, personality, and learning style. It is important to understand and respect that while building the collective effort toward achieving mutual goals.

- Another executive took a top leadership position in one of the health system's large service areas, which had seen major financial losses. She worked hard to correct financial problems and improve quality of service delivery. However, she received feedback that she was not a good fit and that the organization was not ready for someone like her. Eventually, she was fired. It was her first major career setback.

  This executive recovered by taking a period of reflection to learn from the situation and work on her inner development to maintain a positive attitude, self-respect, and self-esteem. She said, "I always know that whatever I left is always going to be better than when I came in. . . . People that know you will give you comfort, compassion, and support." Another reflection on being fired was that the "nature of taking positions of risk is that there will always be a setback. . . . I don't think there is a clear path to up." The next move was to a top executive position at another medical center that was part of a large system. **Key points:** Learn as much as possible about corporate politics, organizational culture, and previous leadership approaches in new positions. Determine whether your leadership style and approaches "fit" the organizational cultural and political dynamics. If possible, learn this information before taking the position. Adapt as needed, without losing sight of who you are, your values, and what you stand for as a person and as a leader.

Key Themes for Rebounding from Mistakes and Setbacks

These examples demonstrate that it is possible to rebound from mistakes and career setbacks. Reflecting on a setback, one executive said, "I went from having one of the most challenging, negative periods in my career to . . . one of the most challenging, positive growth, and developmental periods in my career." In all of these cases, the executives rebounded by reflecting on their values and on what they learned from these experiences, and by using the lessons learned to move forward with more clarity about themselves and their career path.

When the going gets tough on the career journey, life and work can be difficult. The executives in this study navigated difficult people and situations with a strong sense of mission and values. These positive values and personal qualities, along with a focus on providing quality care, were both the foundation and the compass for finding their way through tough circumstances. The strength to cope came from within and from mentors, coaches, colleagues, family, friends, and other trusted advisers. Inner qualities and good relationships provide stable ground during times of great uncertainty and instability.

No matter how rough the path became, these executives were resilient and persevered. The ability to bounce back and stay the course proved to be invaluable. The good news is that they all recovered and continued to advance on the executive path.

KEY LESSONS

- Maintain credibility with performance, results, and positive relationships.

- Focus on what is most important—the reason the organization exists and purpose of the work.

- Maintain a positive frame of mind.

- Adapt as the situation requires, but do not lose sight of your values and self-respect.

- Assess the situation and whether it offers sufficient social and political capital to succeed.

- Recognize what you can and cannot control.

- Stick with challenging people and situations long enough to achieve results and determine when it is a no-win situation.

- Expect to be treated with respect and give constructive feedback to those who are not respectful.

- Seek support to cope with the psychological and emotional effects of challenging bosses, difficult situations, and mistakes and setbacks.

- Engage in activities that facilitate mental, emotional, and physical well-being, such as exercise, yoga, meditation, and healthy diet.

- View all challenges, mistakes, and setbacks as learning opportunities. Apply the lessons learned to accelerate your growth.

EXECUTIVE COMMENTARY

"It takes courage to express concerns in difficult situations, particularly when ethical boundaries are in question. Think about your options, understanding the risk of speaking up. Know your boundaries and don't push them beyond doing what is right. When you know you have made the right decision, you can rest in that."

"As a leader, one of the biggest lessons is realizing when you are wrong. It takes courage to be able to say, 'I made a mistake and need to regroup.' It takes the same courage to say that to your team and ask for their help."

—Deborah Addo, CEO, Inova Loudoun Hospital

"During difficult times, there is value in reaching out to your informal board of advisers (mentors and coaches) for support and guidance."

"There are a lot of career setbacks that don't show up on the résumé, such as promotions that you did not attain. The most important thing you can do is to develop a healthy perspective on those setbacks and not become distracted or discouraged."

—Dr. Sachin H. Jain, MD, MBA, President and CEO, CareMore Health

"It is important to turn a crisis into an opportunity. Instead of complaining and blaming, find solutions and work collaboratively. See a different angle of the crisis and make it a win–win for all involved."

—Dr. Ram Raju, MD, MBA, Senior Vice President and
Community Health Investment Officer,
Northwell Health

Reflection and Action

Think about the tough situations that you have experienced in the past:

- What significant lessons did you learn?
- What did you learn about yourself and leadership?
- How did you apply the lessons learned?

Think about the tough situations that you are experiencing now:

- What lessons are you learning?
- What are you learning about yourself and your leadership style?
- What will you do to apply those lessons?
- What will you do to engage a circle of support?

CHAPTER 9

Leadership Makes the Difference

As you read this chapter on leadership, I invite you to reflect on your own leadership. What does leadership mean to you? How has leadership made a difference in the positions you have held? What role has leadership played in your career advancement? The last two questions were asked throughout the interviews about each position on the executive path.

Before sharing what I learned about leadership from the executives interviewed for this study, I think it is helpful to have a context for understanding their experiences. In healthcare, leadership has almost become cliché because it has been talked and written about so much. This does not diminish the importance of leadership for addressing the critical issues that healthcare organizations face today. Rather, it indicates how much leadership is needed. Leadership remains a key factor that determines how populations are served by healthcare providers and how stakeholders work together to create healthy communities.

There are so many definitions of leadership, however. What leadership means is the subject of ongoing debate and discovery. This confusion about what leadership means is complicated by the fact that the term "leadership" is often used interchangeably with "management." I want to clarify the difference, so that as we discuss the leadership demonstrated by the executives in this study, we are really describing their leadership rather than their management capabilities. Leadership is what made them stand out among many other capable managers.

THE DIFFERENCE BETWEEN LEADERSHIP AND MANAGEMENT

Countless books and articles have been written about leadership and management. Leadership scholar Dr. John P. Kotter (1990) in his seminal book *A Force for Change: How Leadership Differs from Management* provides useful definitions. He clearly differentiates leadership and management in terms of their primary functions while acknowledging the similarities between the two practices.

Kotter (1990, 6) compares management and leadership using the example of creating an agenda for change. Management focuses on planning and budgeting. Detailed steps, time frames, and financial resources are developed to achieve results. Management also involves organizing the structure, staffing, lines of authority and delegation, policies and procedures, and systems required to implement the agenda. Controlling and problem-solving are important activities for monitoring results and making adjustments. These actions create order and consistency in outcomes. Management tends to focus on maintaining the status quo and stability. However, in today's ever-changing, complex, and turbulent healthcare environment, this has become more challenging.

What is leadership, according to Kotter? Leadership develops a vision for the future and the change strategies needed to achieve that vision. People must be aligned with the vision and committed to implementing the strategies. They need to be motivated and inspired to work through the challenges that inevitably will arise in any major change process. Mobilizing and inspiring people to contribute their ideas to the collective effort to achieve a shared vision differentiates leadership from management.

Clearly, both management and leadership are necessary to be effective. They are "intertwined constructs" (Riggio 2017, 276), not dichotomous. My doctoral dissertation research looked at the relationship between transactional and transformational CEO leadership and hospital performance. Transactional leadership is aligned with management in that it focuses on the transactions that leaders engage in with followers to accomplish the work (Bass and Riggio 2006). For example, executing projects in a timely manner in exchange for recognition and reward for performance is transactional leadership. On the other hand, in transformational leadership, leaders inspire, motivate, and empower followers to become leaders in the collective effort to achieve a shared vision and goals (Bass and Riggio 2006; Burns 1978). The results of my dissertation study indicated that a balance of both transactional (capable management) and transformational leadership behaviors by CEOs led to a positive difference in their hospitals (Dixon 1997, 1998).

Kotter (1990) makes the point that not everyone who is in a leadership position is a leader. Most of us have had experiences that confirm this assertion. What facilitated career advancement for the executives in this book was that they demonstrated leadership well before they were in positions that required it. Before we take a closer look at the types of leadership that made a difference, let's examine a definition of leadership that is specific to healthcare.

HEALTHCARE DEFINITION OF LEADERSHIP

The Healthcare Leadership Alliance (HLA), a consortium of six professional membership organizations, including the American College of Healthcare Executives (ACHE), has identified five competency domains that are common among healthcare managers (HLA 2010; Stefl 2008). Competencies are defined as clusters of knowledge, skills, and abilities that transcend organizational settings. Considerable research forms the basis of the domains. The leadership domain is central and interconnects with the four other domains: communication and relationship management, professionalism, knowledge of the healthcare environment, and business skills and knowledge. Leadership is defined as the "ability to inspire individual and organizational excellence, create a shared vision and successfully manage change to attain the organization's strategic ends and successful performance" (Stefl 2008, 364).

This competency model is the basis for the "ACHE Healthcare Executive 2019 Competencies Assessment Tool." In this tool, the leadership domain encompasses leadership skills and behavior, organizational climate and culture, communicating vision, and managing change (HLA and ACHE 2019). Each of these competencies is further defined with specific skills and behaviors. This definition of leadership and related competencies are closely aligned with Kotter's definition and with transformational leadership.

Now that we have a context for understanding the meaning of leadership, let's explore how leadership had a significant influence on the career trajectories of the study participants.

LEADERSHIP MAKES THE DIFFERENCE

Leadership was further defined by the executives in this study as they discussed how they advanced in their careers. The leadership competencies that made a difference are not new or different from the definitions given in the previous section and that we know from experience. Rather, we are learning from racially and ethnically diverse leaders who are often not included in leadership research and books. Leadership scholars have not often addressed the diversity of leaders in terms of race, ethnicity, gender, or sexual orientation (Eagly and Chin 2010). This study presents an opportunity to include them in the research of understanding leadership. It is particularly relevant, since according to the US Census Bureau the population is becoming increasingly diverse.

According to a focus group study of diverse leaders, participants recognized that the multiple dimensions of identity, such as race/ethnicity and gender, do influence leadership practice (Chin, Desormeaux, and Sawyer 2016). The researchers used an intersectionality lens, considering the different dimensions of identity as interrelated and operating simultaneously (Crenshaw 1989). For this study, it is understood that the racial/ethnic identity of the executives is interconnected with their lived experiences of how their leadership influenced their career advancement. Their identities are embedded in the responses.

THE BEGINNINGS OF LEADERSHIP

In the early stages of their careers, these executives held positions that required a higher degree of management skills. They received recognition and rewards for their excellent execution of projects and tasks. While working in this capacity, they began to exhibit leadership by identifying changes that would make their departments more effective. They demonstrated the ability to mobilize people for positive action to attain collective goals. Leadership became a signature of their ability to take on increasingly broader responsibilities in more complex organizational settings.

In the process, they became more than just capable managers. They inspired larger groups of people to work as teams to achieve goals across multiple functions and organizational groups. Leadership made them stand out among their colleagues and fostered their career advancement.

12 KEY LEADERSHIP COMPETENCIES

In many of the stories that the executives shared about their experiences on the executive path, leadership competencies were a common theme. This section discusses the 12 competencies that were mentioned consistently when the study participants were asked what leadership competencies helped them complete a project, lead a change process, achieve goals in the positions they held, or attain a promotion. These competencies do not describe the full scope of leadership for each study participant. These executives are different people with diverse experiences and leadership approaches that embody who they are as individuals. However, they shared several leadership competencies that contributed to their success along their journeys.

I want to clarify the term "competency." I use it to indicate that in each domain, an array of interrelated knowledge, skills, abilities, and qualities enable the performance of leadership. The research did not seek to describe all aspects of each competency, but rather to gain a general understanding of what type of leadership influenced these executives' career trajectories.

As you review these leadership competencies and reflect on your own, I would like to offer a different lens to look through. The competencies are listed for ease of reading, but that is not the best way to understand them. When you see leadership in action, you do not see a list. Effective leadership performance is not about executing an ordered list of competencies. It is more like a performing art (Vaill 1989). These competencies are performed in combination with each other, and they are interrelated.

Executives determine which leadership behaviors will work in a particular situation given competing priorities. Just as in art, such as in a dance or an impressionist painting, it takes creativity and intuition to discern which move to make or how to create a picture of the future for the organization so that people at all levels will embrace it. Leadership is a process of figuring out what works and what does not work in service to mission. When you read about these leadership competencies, think of them in connection to the positive personal qualities that you read about in chapter 3. They go hand in hand. The whole person leads.

Any one of the leadership competencies could be the subject of a chapter itself, but for the purposes of this book, they are briefly described as the executives in the study talked about them and in the context of the factors that influenced their advancement to the C-suite. Hopefully, you will gain enough insight to want to explore them in depth from the perspective of your own career journey or as a mentor, coach, or sponsor.

Emotional Intelligence

Most of us are familiar with the meaning of emotional intelligence and its relationship to effective leadership. According to psychologist and science journalist Dr. Daniel Goleman (2000), emotional intelligence means managing one's self and relationships effectively through four basic capabilities: self-awareness, self-management, social awareness, and social skill. His research indicates that emotional intelligence is a leadership competency that is related to performance.

In the interviews, the executives expressed that they were continually working on and mindful of their emotional intelligence. Several study participants explicitly used the term "emotional intelligence," while others referred to it implicitly in their own words. For example, one executive whom I call Ralph said, "I think I displayed a reasonable level of emotional intelligence and figured out how to manage through circumstances with people with different personalities." In another instance, Mary talked about her ability to self-reflect and adapt her leadership behaviors.

Similarly, Paula reflected often and understood her strengths and weaknesses, which enabled her to continuously enhance her leadership capabilities. Finally, Calvin described how he had gained a "sharpened awareness about emotional intelligence, giving him the tools and insights to know himself and know the personal side that would contribute to the professional side." This comment sums up the collective thinking of these executives about the importance of emotional intelligence.

Based on the stories that these executives told, I want to expand the definition of emotional intelligence to include mettle—that is, the ability to cope with difficulties with strength of character and perseverance. These executives developed the mettle to manage multiple competing priorities across sometimes conflicting boundaries. It was mettle that enabled the executives who experienced racial/ethnic or gender microaggressions to navigate those situations with dignity and integrity. Mettle enabled those who were the only person of color or woman in the room to manage those situations effectively. They had the strength of character to stick with the job and to achieve in the face of all kinds of challenges. For this reason, I regard mettle as an underlying characteristic of emotional intelligence for these leaders.

Learning Mindfully

Learning mindfully means that you are fully attentive to what you are learning in the moment. The ability to learn mindfully in the midst of action and to be open to learning at all times was a consistent theme expressed in the interviews. "Mindful" means consciously and intentionally learning.

Mindfulness was described in a variety of ways by the study participants. They often talked about lessons learned and learning moments. They spoke of "learning how to manage up" and "learning the latest process and quality improvement tools and methodologies." One executive said, "I had to learn how to get work done with groups of people and teams," while another explained, "We all learned from each other." Others talked about "learning to deal with adversity."

Calvin described learning in a way that echoed what others said: "Really understanding what you know and understanding better what you don't know; then you ask questions and cover those things you need answers to because you don't know; the third piece is making sure you are doing it the right way." In addition to these specific comments about learning, many of the executives spoke implicitly of learning. Openness to learning was at the heart of many reflections about their career experiences, relationships, job changes, and mistakes and career setbacks.

Learning mindfully is about more than just being open to learning. These executives demonstrated the ability to learn in moments of action and to adapt their leadership approaches. Learning characterized who they are as leaders. When I was reflecting on leading in moments of action, it dawned on me that a former professor, Dr. Peter Vaill (1996), wrote an entire book titled *Learning as a Way of Being*. Vaill calls this kind of learning "leaderly learning," meaning that the process of learning is going on all the time in executive life and leadership is learning (Vaill 1996, 127). This characterized the executives I interviewed. They were "leaderly" learners. Not only were they learning all the time, but they consciously leveraged that learning to develop their leadership, which enhanced their progression on the executive path.

Developing and Maintaining Relationships

The importance of relationships cannot be emphasized enough. This is why an entire chapter of this book (chapter 4) is dedicated to its value and impact on career advancement. It is also a competency in that developing and maintaining relationships with people at all levels and directions in the organization, as well as with internal and external stakeholders, is central to leadership.

Relationship management is understanding the interrelationships and interdependencies among people inside and outside of the organization. It is the ability to facilitate these interactions in a way that promotes the teamwork required to achieve quality-centered goals and service excellence. Organizational change efforts depend on creating positive and productive relationships with all people and not losing sight of the front line.

The study participants learned this early in their careers. They all talked about the value of getting to know people and developing strong and trusting relationships. One of Alvin's stories, about becoming a new leader in a hospital, mirrored those of the other executives. One of Alvin's first priorities when he began as a hospital top executive in a health system was "getting to know the people." For example, he reflected on how he "got to know every physician and would meet them in the physicians' lounge early in the morning." Further, he walked the units twice a day to get to know the hospital's people and work processes. In this way, Alvin not only developed relationships as a new leader but also learned what needed to change to build a culture and work environment in which people would be committed to the hospital's mission and vision.

This example highlights the importance of relationship management, which was fundamental for Alvin's accomplishments and those of the other executives. Building and sustaining relationships was key for successful leadership and instrumental in their career trajectories.

Effective Communication

Effective communication is another leadership competency that helped advance these executives' careers. But communication is not to be taken for granted. So often, ineffective communication ruins relationships and derails the most well-thought-out change initiatives. These executives began developing communication skills early in their careers. As they took on increasing responsibilities and managed the complexity of working across multiple boundaries, they recognized the importance of continuing to develop effective communication skills.

Several types of communication in the organizational leadership context made a difference. These include verbal communication skills, such as being able to articulate a message clearly; interpersonal communication skills, including the ability to have meaningful conversations by actively listening individually and in groups; written communication skills; and nonverbal communication skills, meaning the unspoken cues and messages conveyed to others through body language. Time and again, communication was key to maintaining high performance and achieving results.

All of the executives expressed the importance of being highly visible to staff and using multiple forms of communication to reach them. Alvin said, "A good leader is chief communicator," and he talked about how he worked on being a credible messenger. He also talked about the importance of communicating across disciplines and with multiple stakeholders. Reflecting on her success with transformational change in several organizations, Lois indicated that frequent communication was a significant factor. Emily described the value of communication skills no matter the audience. Mary said, "I was able to communicate up and down the ladder; when I walk around, I just talk to everyone and ask them what they are doing." Further, she shared that she could talk with the physicians. Ralph thought that "communicating a positive tone is very important."

Paula emphasized active listening. Cheryl's thinking was in line with Paula's in that she, too, considered listening to be essential. She stressed the importance of "robust conversation in which everyone contributes" and "listening to all the people to hear their concerns to see how to address them." Bob reflected on his ability to listen to what people want and learning from them, which allowed him to stay in touch with what people need to do their jobs and fulfill organizational goals. He considered it as one of his key strengths.

According to these executives, the ability to communicate in multiple forms with multiple stakeholders at all levels, both internally and externally, was central to their advancement to the C-suite. The ability to engage in interpersonal communications with people to understand what is on their minds and in their hearts is the essence of leadership. Leadership is about working with others to attain common goals. Communication enables that to happen.

Collaboration

Collaboration is the process of working together to achieve a goal or to create something, such as an innovative care delivery model. Collaboration also can be a negotiation strategy. As these executives described their careers, the ability to collaborate with others was another key contributor to success on their journeys. Their collaboration was often focused within a hospital, working with departments and divisions earlier in their careers. As they honed their collaboration skills through practice and feedback from colleagues and mentors, they took on broader leadership responsibilities. This required collaboration across multiple organizational boundaries in health systems, often with community and statewide partners and stakeholders. For some, collaboration with colleagues in healthcare associations played an essential role in decision-making about healthcare issues nationally.

Many of the executives described themselves as collaborative leaders. Sarah reflected on her success as a collaborator: "I think above all it has to be [a] collaborator, someone who is willing to be part of the team and willing to figure out how that all comes together." She continued to say, "As we look at healthcare in general and the direction healthcare is moving in, [the] people in the future that will be successful are collaborators." Paula thought that "learning how to bring people from disparate points of view together to make decisions to move the organization forward" was important for her effectiveness as a leader. These quotes are representative of the other comments made about collaboration. The ability to collaborate is a major contributor to success on the executive path.

Engagement of People at All Levels

Engagement is related to people skills but takes it to another level. It is a competency because it involves a combination of knowledge, skills, and abilities such as communication, collaboration, and relationship management. A 2017 Gallup survey defined engaged employees as those who are involved, enthusiastic, and committed to their work. Leadership is required to achieve this level of engagement. Innovation and transformation of delivery systems to meet external demands and improve quality and cost-efficiency cannot happen without it. These executives described how important it was for them to reach people at all levels, not forgetting about the frontline staff.

Tom shared one of his biggest lessons: "You don't tell people what to do; you try to engage their hearts and . . . sense of professionalism." Similarly, Sarah talked about her approach: "It's always been that I'm never going to ask someone to do something I don't do; I was not seen as the suit walking in; I was one of them." She never lost her connection with the frontline staff. In the same vein, Mary said, "Engaging people on all levels in the process of change" made a difference in the culture change efforts that she had led. And Cheryl, as she reflected on her success in completing several major projects, indicated that the engagement of people up and down the line made her success possible. In several transformational change processes in different organizations, Lois indicated that she kept this question top of mind: "How do you generate excitement and engagement?"

These are just a few examples from the stories told during the interviews. The executives all believed in and demonstrated the value of inclusion and engagement in their leadership. It is important to note that they were not just giving lip service to engagement as the latest leadership platitude—they really meant it. Their leadership success reflected their ability to do it well.

Team Development

"Team" is another a term that has become a cliché. It is often used—and sometimes misused—to suggest that all groups are teams. But calling a group a team does not make it so. In their classic book *The Wisdom of Teams*, Jon Katzenbach and Douglas Smith (1993, 45) define a team as "a small number of people with complementary skills who are committed to a common purpose, performance goals, and approach for which they hold themselves mutually accountable." They go further, indicating that in a high-performing team, people actually care and are concerned about each other's personal growth. While many books have been written and studies conducted on teams, this definition remains relevant today. The executives in this study were really talking about teams and their significance for effective leadership.

All of the leadership stories that were shared spoke to how instrumental team development was for developing high-performing hospitals and health systems and health service organizations. These executives were successful because they learned how to do this well. For example, Tom said, "An effective team isn't about just competency. It's about value systems, temperaments, personality styles, and traits. . . . It's about creating a patchwork quilt of different learning styles, different communication systems, [and] different belief systems so you don't get too much groupthink."

Tom's words are representative of the collective experiences with building real teams and elevating performance as a result. A significant lesson that the executives shared was the importance of leadership in creating an environment and culture in which teams can thrive. Team development is another essential factor for success on the executive path.

Leading with Vision

One executive, Bob, described himself as a visionary and an innovator: "For me, the most important role is to set the vision for the organization." His perspective on leading with vision was shared by the other executives. They spoke about vision in different ways. Here are examples that mirror the collective wisdom:

- "I had to learn how to get work done with groups of people [and] teams, and lead people through the vision. . . . I painted a picture of the future."
- Asking the team routinely, "What are the decisions we are going to have to make to position us for the future?"

The executives also discussed the alignment of the vision with mission and values. Tom said, "First and foremost, you create mission, vision, and values alignment." He talked about the need to align staff with goals and objectives and the importance of accountability to achieve those goals and objectives. Earlier, Tom talked about doing this by "engaging their hearts and own sense of professionalism." In doing so, people will more likely align with mission and vision. Ralph also talked about the importance of alignment: "Alignment is a core construct of my leadership tenet."

A significant leadership factor for all the interviewees was that they articulated a vision for the future in alignment with the mission and values of the organizations they worked for during their careers. And importantly, they gained the shared commitment of people to work toward achieving it. This is not easy, and it takes a combination of all of the leadership competencies to make it happen.

Leading and Managing Organizational Change

In today's healthcare organizations, transformational change is at the center of the work. Change is a constant, whether in population health, health information technology, digital integration, innovative delivery models, telehealth, improving the quality of care and patient safety, transitioning to value-based care, closing the gap in healthcare disparities, or other efforts to disrupt dysfunctional systems to achieve better health systems. This is the heart of healthcare leadership.

For this reason, leading and managing change was a significant theme in the interviews. Every move on the executive path journey involved organizational change. The leadership competencies described here worked together to accomplish change. All of the leaders talked a great deal about understanding organizational culture in recognition of the critical role that it plays in successful transformations.

Paula talked about her leadership as she moved to different hospitals within a health system. She believed that "understanding cultural differences between hospitals and learning to navigate it" was crucial for her leadership. Further, she reflected on how this understanding helped her shape the kind of culture she wanted to create. Similarly, Sarah also spoke about culture change and shared an example of an experience that allowed her to build the culture that she wanted with the team. In addition, both Paula and Mary shared the value of learning and applying process redesign and Lean Six Sigma approaches to change strategies. It is important to note that they learned these processes as executive leaders and did not just delegate implementation to their staff.

Organizational turnarounds were significant change initiatives that the majority of the interviewees were responsible for leading. They made learning the organizational culture a top priority, which helped facilitate successful culture change in those organizations.

Leading and managing transformational change was pivotal for these executives' career mobility.

Bridge Building

Hospitals and health systems are large and loosely knitted together so that they can better serve communities in various locations. They function as a complex network of organizational entities that need to collaborate to accomplish goals such as achieving population health and implementing innovative approaches to care delivery. As healthcare organizations recognize the social determinants of health and their critical role in the well-being of diverse populations and communities, building bridges across organizational boundaries such as housing, transportation, and access to nutritious food becomes critical.

In addition, new partnerships such as CVS Health/Aetna and Cigna/Express Scripts and alliances such as Amazon, Berkshire Hathaway, and JPMorgan Chase are competing with traditional healthcare systems to disrupt and transform care delivery models, enhance access, and reduce costs. As the complexity of working with nontraditional alliances increases, so does the likelihood of conflicting priorities and leadership approaches to achieve mutual aims. This makes bridge building a crucial leadership competency.

You might wonder how this is different from relationship management and collaboration. Both of these competencies are necessary to work effectively in complex healthcare organizations. The executives in this study developed connections and linkages by focusing on mutual goals, negotiating conflicting viewpoints, and working to collaboratively bridge the gaps to achieving them. As bridge builders, they acted as facilitators of crucial conversations, which are the foundation for making vital decisions. They built trust through their authenticity and genuine focus on doing what is right for the collective good. It is easy to see that to be an effective bridge builder requires using all of the other leadership competencies. These executives succeeded because they knew how to be bridge builders.

Political Acumen

The ability to navigate organizational politics was quite clear in the stories that the study participants shared. They began to develop that ability early in their careers, sometimes by making mistakes because of their naiveté about the power of organizational politics. Organizational politics is difficult to understand and often difficult to recognize because it is not always visible and frequently is subsumed in the informal organization. The informal organization is the network of relationships and influence that are not represented on formal organizational charts. Organizational politics has been defined as the use of influence strategies to enhance personal or organizational interests (Jarrett 2017). Political acumen has been defined as the ability to "accurately perceive and judge the formal and informal influences that shape decision making" (Andreatta 2013).

One of the study participants described political acumen as "seeing the currents before stepping in the water." This metaphorical description implies that seeing is perceiving, observing, and understanding how decisions are made and who influences that process. In the same vein, Paula noted the importance of being "observant [of] the circumstances you are in until you have the power and authority to shape [them]."

Observing what is seen and heard is easier than observing what is not seen and not heard. That is the position that minorities often find themselves in, because they may not be included in informal networks and conversations. The executives in this study were able to develop political acumen. They did so not only by observing but also by developing rich relationships with people within their organizations, so that they were included in both formal and informal organizational networks.

To "see the currents before stepping in the water" means they were tuned in and able to make connections among individuals and groups so that they could understand the best ways to intervene. They became influencers in decision-making. It is clear that political acumen directly impacts leadership effectiveness. Political mistakes, as several of the study participants learned, can undermine the most well-intentioned and otherwise skilled leader. Political acumen influenced the career trajectories of these executives.

Financial and Business Acumen

It may be stating the obvious to say healthcare is a business, but nonetheless, it is important to emphasize. That is the reason financial and business acumen is essential to executive leadership. ACHE's "2017 Hospital CEO Survey on Employment Contracts and Performance Reviews: Incentive Payments" studied the factors considered in determining executives' incentive pay (ACHE 2018). It showed that financial performance was the number-one factor in determining incentive pay, as reported by 69 percent of CEOs from all hospital types. The executives in this study understood this and made astute financial and business decisions.

Knowledge, skills, and abilities associated with financial and business acumen had to be developed in most cases. This was particularly true for those with clinical backgrounds who did not have finance and business courses in their degree programs. They developed financial and business acumen through a combination of learning on the job and obtaining additional education. In these cases, they learned quickly how departmental or division budgets affected the overall financial management of the hospital. This understanding is essential not only for effective job performance but also for advancement.

As these executives progressed to higher levels of responsibility, financial and business acumen was even more crucial for their leadership. As Alvin said, there are "two bottom lines: one is to do good—taking care of people, patients, and staff—and one is do well as good stewards of financial resources." Joseph agreed, indicating that one of the contributors to his success was having strong accounting and finance skills. He pointed out, "You need to be strong in both relational and transactional capabilities." He described himself in this way: "I'm a steward of someone's investment, be it a public or private hospital." Mary explained that "strong financial skills [are] the only way you are going to be successful." She emphasized the importance of financial skills without minimizing the equal importance of people and engagement skills, which she also felt were her strengths. Describing being asked to lead a major organizational turnaround, Lois noted that "one of the first things is to study and become educated on the financial end of things." These comments are representative of the collective thinking in the research. Financial and business acumen is a requisite competency for career advancement.

IN CONCLUSION

The 12 interrelated leadership competencies, together with the positive personal qualities discussed in chapter 3, facilitated advancement to the C-suite for the executives in this study. Another way to understand them is to use the Center for Creative Leadership's organizing framework for levels of leadership: leading self, leading others, and leading the organization (Van Velsor, McCauley, and Ruderman 2010; see exhibit 9.1). The ways of leading do not function separately, but rather work together in action. There are other leadership competencies and factors that influenced the career trajectories of the study participants. But these competencies were mentioned consistently by all

EXHIBIT 9.1: Leadership Competencies

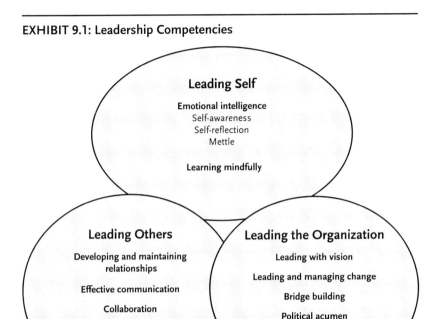

Leading Self

Emotional intelligence
Self-awareness
Self-reflection
Mettle

Learning mindfully

Leading Others

Developing and maintaining
relationships

Effective communication

Collaboration

Engagement

Team development

Leading the Organization

Leading with vision

Leading and managing change

Bridge building

Political acumen

Finance/business acumen

Source: The organizing framework for the leadership competencies is adapted from the Center for Creative Leadership's (2016) levels of leadership. The competencies are based on this study's results.

of the executives. They made a difference in the organizations in which they worked and facilitated the executives' progression on the executive path.

KEY LESSONS

- Leadership and management are interrelated but different practices.
  - Leadership creates a shared vision to mobilize collective wisdom and action to achieve it.

- Management works with people to plan, organize, and monitor strategies to achieve results. Capable management is the foundation for solid performance.
- An effective balance of capable management and leadership in different organizational situations can influence the career trajectory.

- Leadership that inspires commitment, and that develops and empowers collective leadership, influences successful organizational change.
- The 12 leadership competencies are interrelated and work together to create leadership that makes a difference on the executive path.

EXECUTIVE COMMENTARY

"Leadership is guided by purpose, passion, and authenticity. My purpose and passion are driven by the goal to find out how we can get health equity in this country. This has been the focus of my work on the executive path."

—Dr. Ram Raju, MD, MBA, Senior Vice President
and Community Health Investment Officer,
Northwell Health

"As a leader, I remember this quote by Maya Angelou: 'I've learned that people will forget what you said, people will forget what you did, but people will never forget how you made them feel.' . . . My leadership is not just doing. It's about working with and serving people."

—Denise Brooks-Williams, Senior Vice President
and CEO, North Market,
Henry Ford Health System

"One of the most significant leadership competencies is the ability to work with all types of people at all levels and have meaningful conversations with them."

—Phyllis Wingate, President, Atrium Health–Carolinas HealthCare System, North East

"Leadership is hard but rewarding. Sometimes, when you take three steps forward, a prevailing wind takes you back a step. This is where perseverance comes in."

—Rick L. Stevens, FACHE, President, Christian Hospital

"The people that report to you and the colleagues with whom you work are your partners. Work toward developing collaborative relationships. You can't do these jobs alone."

—Eddie Cruz, MBA, FACHE, Vice President of Operations, Access Community Health Network

---

Reflection and Action

- What do you think about the 12 leadership competencies? Are they relevant for your career journey?

- Are you demonstrating these leadership competencies?

- How would you rate your capability in each leadership competency, on a scale from 1 (lowest) to 5 (highest)?

- What is your leadership development action plan for enhancing your strengths and improving the competencies with the most opportunity for growth? (You may want to refer to the "ACHE Healthcare Executive 2019 Competencies Assessment Tool.")

Note to coaches, mentors, and sponsors: The Reflection and Action process can help guide your work with developmental relationships.

REFERENCES

American College of Healthcare Executives (ACHE). 2018. "2017 Hospital CEO Survey on Employment Contracts and Performance Reviews: Incentive Payments August 2017." Accessed May 30, 2019. www.ache.org/learning-center/research/about-the-field/meeting-challenges/ceo-surveys.

Andreatta, B. 2013. "Developing Political Acumen." Published June 25. www.lynda.com/Business-Skills-tutorials/Developing-political-acumen/122471/139739-4.html.

Bass, B. M., and R. E. Riggio. 2006. *Transformational Leadership*, 2nd ed. Mahwah, NJ: Lawrence Erlbaum.

Burns, J. M. 1978. *Leadership*. New York: Harper & Row.

Center for Creative Leadership. 2016. "The Leadership Development Roadmap: A Guide for Developing Successful Leaders at All Levels." Accessed May 29, 2019. www.ccl.org/wp-content/uploads/2016/09/leader-development-roadmap-center-for-creative-leadership.pdf.

Chin, J. L., L. Desormeaux, and K. Sawyer. 2016. "Making Way for Paradigms of Diversity Leadership." *Consulting Psychology Journal: Practice and Research* 68 (1): 49–71.

Crenshaw, K. 1989. "Demarginalizing the Intersection of Race and Sex: A Black Feminist Critique of Antidiscrimination Doctrine, Feminist Theory, and Antiracist Politics." *University of Chicago Legal Forum* 140: 139–67.

Dixon, D. L. 1998. "The Balanced CEO: A Transformational Leader and a Capable Manager." *Healthcare Forum Journal* 41 (2): 26–29.

———. 1997. "The Relationship Between Chief Executive Leadership (Transactional and Transformational) and Hospital Effectiveness." EdD diss., George Washington University.

Eagly, A. H., and J. L. Chin. 2010. "Diversity and Leadership in a Changing World." *American Psychologist* 65 (3): 216–24.

Gallup. 2017. "Gallup Daily: US Engagement." Accessed May 29, 2019. https://news.gallup.com/poll/180404/gallup-daily-employee-engagement.aspx.

Goleman, D. 2000. "Leadership That Gets Results." *Harvard Business Review* 78 (2): 16–28.

Healthcare Leadership Alliance (HLA). 2010. "Healthcare Leadership Alliance." Accessed May 29, 2019. www.healthcareleadershipalliance.org/directory.htm.

Healthcare Leadership Alliance (HLA) and American College of Healthcare Executives (ACHE). 2019. "ACHE Healthcare Executive 2019 Competencies Assessment Tool." Accessed May 29. www.ache.org/-/media/ache/career-resource-center/competencies_booklet.pdf.

Jarrett, M. 2017. "The 4 Types of Organizational Politics." *Harvard Business Review*. Published April 24. https://hbr.org/2017/04/the-4-types-of-organizational-politics.

Katzenbach, J. R., and D. K. Smith. 1993. *The Wisdom of Teams*. New York: Harper Business.

Kotter, J. P. 1990. *A Force for Change: How Leadership Differs from Management*. New York: Free Press.

Riggio, R. E. 2017. "Management and Leadership." In *The Oxford Handbook of Management*, edited by A. Wilkinson, S. J. Armstrong, and M. Lounsbury, 276–92. Oxford: Oxford University Press.

Stefl, M. E. 2008. "Common Competencies for All Healthcare Managers: The Healthcare Leadership Alliance Model." *Journal of Healthcare Management* 53 (6): 360–72.

Vaill, P. B. 1996. *Learning as a Way of Being: Strategies for Survival in a World of Permanent White Water*. San Francisco: Jossey-Bass.

―――. 1989. *Managing as a Performing Art: New Ideas for a World of Chaotic Change*. San Francisco: Jossey-Bass.

Van Velsor, E., C. D. McCauley, and M. N. Ruderman (eds.). 2010. *The Center for Creative Leadership Handbook of Leadership Development*, 3rd ed. San Francisco: John Wiley & Sons.

CHAPTER 10

Discerning What Matters Most

AFTER READING THE previous chapters, you may be asking yourself these questions: What matters most? What are the most important takeaways? What does all of this mean for me? How can I use this information to help me discern the next phases of my career journey? This chapter will help you reflect on these questions.

DISCERNING WHAT MATTERS MOST:
THE SEVEN ESSENTIALS

Discernment is the process of making judgments based on what you are learning and blending those judgments with your own experience. In essence, it is determining what matters most for your journey and what will make a significant difference in your career path.

The lessons learned from the lived experiences shared in this book all have value; however, there are a few essentials that will help you build a foundation for ongoing growth. I call them "wisdom facilitators." I say this because in practicing the essentials, you will gain experience and knowledge and sharpen your ability to make good judgments. Wisdom will help you to navigate the twists and turns on the executive path. Your direction will likely change, because life is an adventure and no matter how much you plan, you will encounter unknowns that will change your path. If you have a few guides and use your wisdom, you will be better able to manage the complexity of life and career.

The following seven essentials are drawn from the wisdom of the 12 research participants and supported by the executive commentators (see exhibit 10.1). While the wisdom of others provides insights and lessons, it is important to develop your own.

The essentials are not listed in order of priority. They work together synergistically: More can be achieved by understanding and embracing the interrelationships among them. They are not steps on a ladder up to the C-suite or executive level, but rather guides and facilitators for your career path discernment and practice.

- Know "you" and work toward being the best person you can be.
- Develop and maintain positive relationships through authenticity, collaboration, and teamwork.
- Perform and work hard, remembering to develop emotional, social, political, and cultural competence.
- Earn sponsors and seek mentors.
- Learn mindfully and continuously.
- Expand your comfort zone.
- Practice leadership from the heart of your goodness with a focus on mission.

Practicing the seven essentials provides a foundation for using the other lessons in this book.

PRACTICING THE ESSENTIALS

A useful process for discernment and developing the wisdom needed to make good decisions is inquiry and reflection. What follows are suggestions for self-inquiry and reflection that will help

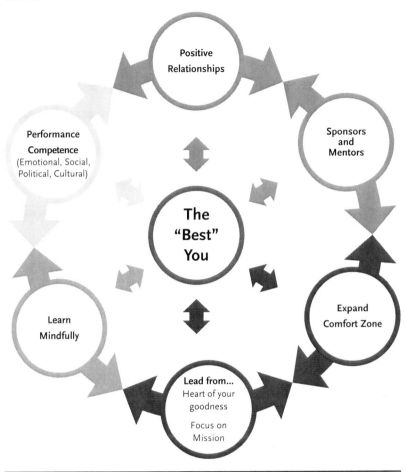

you practice the essentials. It is important to note the difference between action and practice. Action is a process of doing something to achieve a goal, whereas a practice is performed regularly to acquire, improve, or maintain capability and capacity. The two concepts are related, but the difference is that a practice is performed routinely—it is an ongoing process that is embedded in your leadership development. Navigating your career and life journey involves engaging in practices that will enable you to continuously improve and achieve your goals.

The following questions are intended to facilitate inquiry and reflection about where you are now and what you need to do to enhance your growth.

Know "you" and work toward being the best person you can be

- What are your values?
- What are you really passionate about?
- What is your mission?
- What are your positive personal qualities? Which ones do you need to nurture and develop?
- What are your strengths? What are your opportunities for improvement?
- What is your personality type? What does that knowledge tell you about how you prefer to work, your interactions with people and groups, and your leadership?
- What do you need to do to strengthen your self-esteem and self-confidence?
- What do you need to do to be the best person you can be?
- What do you need to do to maintain a balanced and healthy life?

Action: Reflect, Discern, Practice

Develop and maintain positive relationships through authenticity, collaboration, and teamwork

- What is the current state of your relationships? Which ones need nurturing?
- What are you doing to develop genuine relationships?
- What types of relationships do you need to develop to enhance yourself as a professional and as a person?

- How could you become a better collaborator, teammate, and team leader?
- What would help you build relationship capital?

Action: Reflect, Discern, Practice

Perform and develop emotional, social, political, and cultural competence

- What do you need to do to improve your performance? How can you make a positive difference? Think about small actions that can have a big impact.
- Do you need to work harder or smarter? What changes do you need to make?
- What would enrich your emotional competence—not only by developing self-awareness, but also by engaging in the inner work that develops your mettle?
- What would enhance your social competence? For example, how could you improve your ability to interact and develop relationships with people who are different from you?
- What would improve your political competence? For example, how could you better understand and navigate power and influence in informal networks?
- What would enrich your cultural competence?
  - What would enrich your capability to appreciate and work with diverse groups of people with different racial and ethnic backgrounds?
  - What would enhance your capability to better understand and work effectively in different organizational cultures?

Action: Reflect, Discern, Practice

Earn sponsors and seek mentors

- What are you doing to earn sponsors?
  - Are you cultivating genuine relationships with colleagues and potential sponsors?
  - What are you doing to demonstrate that you are worth the risk of sponsoring?
  - Are willing to say yes to new assignments that will challenge you?
  - Are you volunteering for projects, committees, and teams that will enhance your visibility?
  - Are you developing innovative approaches that will help achieve the organization's mission and vision?
  - Do the people who matter know about your accomplishments and potential?
  - Are you communicating your career goals to people who can help you achieve them?
- What are you doing to seek mentors who can provide support, guidance, and advice and share experiences?

Action: Reflect, Discern, Practice

Learn mindfully and continuously

- What would help you become attentive to learning in moments of action?
- What do you need to do to be more intentional and mindful about learning?
- What would enrich your learning mindset to embrace every experience as a learning opportunity?

- What are you doing to put learning into practice—that is, to integrate learning into your work and life?

Action: Reflect, Discern, Practice

Expand your comfort zone

- What can you do to develop a sense of ease and to minimize anxiety in new, difficult, and challenging situations?
- What are you doing to become comfortable being uncomfortable?
  - For example, if you are the only or one of a few minorities in your organization, department or division, or work-related social setting, what will help develop your capacity to be comfortable?
- What would enable you to become more comfortable taking risks, such as taking on a new assignment or positions or changing your position or organization?
- What would help you to become comfortable initiating new relationships, especially with diverse people or people who are different from you?

Action: Reflect, Discern, Practice

Practice leadership from the heart of your goodness with a focus on mission

- What is the heart or center of your goodness? What actions and behaviors demonstrate your goodness?
- What is the purpose for your leadership in healthcare? What is your mission? What is your vision?

- What can you do to integrate the heart of your goodness into your leadership?
- What will help you lead from the heart of your goodness in the midst of challenges and constant change?

Action: Reflect, Discern, Practice

MAKING THIS PROCESS WORK FOR YOU

The key to making this process meaningful for you is to make a commitment to integrate it into your personal and leadership development. Engaging in the process of reflection, discernment, and practice is a way to develop the habit of continuous learning and self-discovery and turn the lessons from this book into routine practices. Consider doing the following to get the most benefit:

- Set aside a specific time for individual leadership and personal development reflection.
  - Tips: Start small—for example, 20 minutes per week.
  - Put it on your calendar.
  - You can do this anywhere, but it works best where there are minimal distractions.
- Write down your thoughts and ideas in a leadership and personal development reflection journal. The journal can be online or on paper. What is important is that you create a space to write down your reflections.
- Conduct a self-assessment based on your reflection and discernment to determine your current capability and capacity for each essential.
- Based on your assessment, identify the essentials for which you have the most opportunity for growth. Develop SMART (specific, measurable, achievable, realistic, and time-bound) goals for the areas you want to strenghten and in which you want to improve.

- Identify a trusted adviser (or advisers) whom you believe can help you with this process. Consider mentors, coaches, sponsors, and colleagues.
  - Engage advisers for this purpose. Communicate your intentions and what you need from them to achieve your goals.
  - Work with them to develop a plan to attain each goal.
  - Determine how you will monitor progress on your plan.
  - Ask for positive and negative feedback. Remember, specific negative feedback is an invaluable teacher.
- Develop a circle of personal support. Beyond professional mentors, coaches, and sponsors, a circle of personal support may include friends, family, significant others such as spouses and partners, counselors, and faith communities that care about you and want to see you succeed. Your circle of personal support lifts you higher. Enough cannot be said about the value of meaningful conversations in which you can relax and share from your heart, trusting that the listeners are there for you.

This process is focused on the seven essentials. Hopefully, you will use it for other lessons that have significant meaning and relevance for you. Even though your specific goals are time-bound for this phase of the process, career and leadership development is ongoing.

USE YOUR WISDOM

The wisdom that you are developing will help you clarify your career and life mission, vision, and possibilities. Whatever is next for you—whether it is getting on the executive path, continuing on it, or getting off it—what matters most is that you are energized by your passion and living your mission and values.

CHAPTER 11

Closing Thoughts for the Journey

As I close this book, I am thinking about what a privilege it is to share the wisdom of 23 diverse healthcare executives—12 research participants and 11 executive commentators. They are amazing leaders who were willing to give us the gift of their experiences and career and life lessons. I am grateful and humbled by the opportunity to write this book so that you can learn from them.

I would like to share a few closing thoughts based on what I have learned, and continue to learn, about the lived experiences of racially and ethnically diverse professionals on the executive path in healthcare.

The underrepresentation of racial/ethnic and other minorities in the C-suite and executive positions in healthcare has been verified in research and practice. Further, the business case for increasing diversity at the senior executive level is well documented. Yet the challenge of achieving executive diversity that is representative of the increasingly diverse population that healthcare serves continues.

From my perspective as a leadership and organization development educator and consultant, I believe that what we have learned from racial and ethnic minorities who have attained the C-suite will help other minorities attain this goal. And these lessons will assist mentors, sponsors, coaches, teachers, and other professionals who support their leadership and career development. I hope this book, along with all the work that is being done by others in the field, will help. Importantly, I hope that the insights presented in this book will inspire more research, productive actions, and practices that will lead to real results. The opportunity is there for you to do what you can do from your sphere of influence and expertise to make an impact in expanding diversity in healthcare executive leadership.

A CHANGING C-SUITE

If the C-suite is your goal for making an impact in healthcare, some changes may give you more opportunities to do it. New C-suite positions are emerging. An article in *Healthcare Executive* titled "Healthcare Changes and New C-Suite Roles" indicates that healthcare leadership is transforming as complex forces such as value-based care, big data, changing delivery models, and the emergence of private sector corporations disrupt the field (Justice 2018). As a result, C-suite positions such as chief population health management officer, chief innovation officer, chief experience officer, chief transformation officer, chief strategy officer, and chief informatics officer are being created. More will likely develop as the field continues to change. When you think about what backgrounds and types of experiences are needed to attain these positions, there may be some new ideas evolving. What is not likely to change are the lessons and insights about what it takes to reach this leadership level from the executives in this book.

THE C-SUITE IS NOT THE ONLY WAY TO LEAD

Is the C-suite for everyone? Is it the only way to make a difference in healthcare? Do you need to be an executive to effect change where it matters? These are questions that I have pondered, and hope you will, too. The C-suite and executive leadership is not for everyone. It is not the only way to make a difference. There are many ways to serve and have an impact. Leadership can come from anywhere in an organization or community. You do not have to be in the C-suite to be a chief. You can be a chief of making positive significant difference anywhere. And you do not need a title to serve and lead. The title "chief" suggests a leader. A synonym for chief is "champion." A champion is a person who voluntarily takes an extraordinary interest in the implementation and success of a policy, program, project, or product. I would add service to this list of options. In healthcare, there are so many areas in which to be a champion. Based on this thinking, I redefined the C-suite (see exhibit 11.1). According to this definition, the C-suite refers to a champion of significant difference with an unrelenting dedication to doing good using innovative practices for transformational change through the engagement of people's hearts and minds.

EXHIBIT 11.1: The C-Suite Redefined

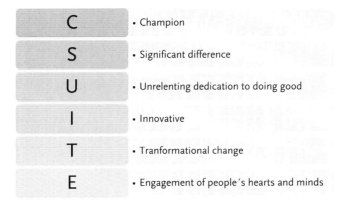

C	• Champion
S	• Significant difference
U	• Unrelenting dedication to doing good
I	• Innovative
T	• Tranformational change
E	• Engagement of people's hearts and minds

You decide how and where you want to lead based on your passion, mission, vision, and values. The process of reflection, discernment, and practice can help guide the decisions you make along your career journey.

I leave you to continue reflecting in the hope that you will move forward and embrace the many possibilities for making a significant difference in healthcare. Whatever you do, live your passion and values with mission in mind. Let the "best you" from the heart of your goodness lead the way.

REFERENCE

Justice, B. 2018. "Healthcare Changes and New C-Suite Roles." *Healthcare Executive* 33 (6): 30–38.

Research Overview

THE UNDERREPRESENTATION OF racially and ethnically diverse professionals in hospital and health system C-suites, particularly at the CEO level, is well documented in the academic and practitioner literature. For example, according to a 2015 study conducted by the Institute for Diversity and Health Equity in collaboration with the Health Research and Educational Trust, "Diversity and Disparities: A Benchmarking Study of U.S. Hospitals," only 9 percent of hospital and health system CEOs belonged to racial/ ethnic minority groups, a figure that remained unchanged from previous studies conducted in 2013 and 2011. Supporting those findings, another study published by the American College of Healthcare Executives in 2015, "A Racial/Ethnic Comparison of Career Attainments in Healthcare Management," indicated that more white men than minority men in the sample identified themselves as CEOs. Similarly, white women held a higher percentage of CEO positions than minority women.

US Census Bureau projections document the changing demographics of the United States, indicating that by 2044, more than half the US population will be part of a minority group (Colby and Ortman 2015). Further, the US Bureau of Labor Statistics' employment projections for 2016–26 indicate that the labor force will continue to become more racially and ethnically diverse. For example, the numbers of Asian and Hispanic/Latino workers are projected to grow faster than the annual average rate from 2016 to 2026, at 2.5 percent and 2.7 percent, respectively (US Bureau of Labor Statistics 2017). The increasing diversity of the US population and workforce underscores the need for culturally competent healthcare organizations and diverse leadership that mirrors the population of healthcare consumers.

A number of studies have focused on the need for cultural competence among hospitals and health systems and the need for leadership diversity (Dansky et al. 2003; Dotson and Nuru-Jeter 2012; Dreachslin 1999, 2007a, 2007b; Dreachslin and Hobby 2008; Dreachslin, Weech-Maldonado, and Dansky 2004; Dreachslin et al. 2017; Flores and Combs 2013). Embedded in this literature is the important role that top executives play in creating a culture of diversity and culturally competent organizations. The evidence is clear that more diverse executive leadership is needed in healthcare (ACHE 2015a, 2015b; Brown 2015; Dolan 2013; Dreachslin and Hobby 2008; Institute for Diversity and Health Equity 2015; Witt/Kieffer 2011).

However, few studies have focused specifically on the role of the CEO in developing diverse and culturally competent hospitals and health systems and the relationship of the CEO with the executive team to achieve this goal (Dreachslin et al. 2017). Many studies of the role of CEOs and top executive teams and how they influence organizational performance have focused on corporations, not healthcare. Several of these studies indicate that CEOs do play a key role in influencing organizational outcomes (Carmeli, Schaubroeck, and Tishler 2011; Finkelstein and Hambrick 1996; Hambrick 2007; Hambrick and Mason 1984; Hambrick and Quigley 2014).

A number of dissertation research studies have also examined the role of CEOs and hospital performance. For example, a study examining the relationship between chief executive leadership (transactional and transformational) and hospital effectiveness suggested that chief executives use both transactional and transformational behaviors directly and indirectly to affect hospital effectiveness through the creation and implementation of strategy, structure, control systems, and distribution of power and core values (Dixon 1997). Specifically, the study found a significant relationship between transformational leadership characteristics (confident leadership and visionary leadership) and patient satisfaction, as measured by The Leadership Profile (TLP) developed by William E. Rosenbach and Marshall Sashkin (Rosenbach, Sashkin, and Harburg 1996).

Based on these studies, it is reasonable to posit that CEOs play a significant role in effecting the organizational development and cultural change needed to create culturally competent organizations (Dreachslin 2007a, 2007b; Dreachslin et al. 2017; Schein 2010). That said, given the body of work on the need for more diversity in the C-suite and what we are learning about the CEO role, it stands to reason that we need to learn more about how to increase the number of racially and ethnically diverse CEOs in hospitals and health systems. There has been scant research on this specific topic and limited research examining how minorities who have reached the CEO position got there (ACHE 2015b; Sexton, Lemak, and Wainio 2014).

MINORITY CEOs AND CAREER ADVANCEMENT

As indicated earlier, few studies have examined the executive career experiences of racially and ethnically diverse professionals, including leadership competencies that facilitate advancement to the C-suite. Leadership research and studies on diverse leaders are fruitful avenues of future study, as the majority of seminal leadership studies do not include racial and ethnic minorities (Eagly and Chin 2010). A limited number of studies have focused on how diverse leaders lead and how their leadership behavior is shaped by the intersection of their racial/ethnic and gender identities (Chin, Desormeaux, and

Sawyer 2016; Crenshaw 1989). And there is a paucity of literature on how leadership has influenced the career advancement of racially and ethnically diverse professionals to the C-suite in healthcare.

Seminal research conducted by David A. Thomas and John J. Gabarro (1999) examined minority executive development and advancement in three for-profit non-healthcare corporations in the United States. These researchers focused on 20 case studies of successful minority executives: 13 African Americans, 4 Asian Americans, and 3 Hispanic/Latino Americans. Women who met the executive criteria were included. The researchers compared these executives' experiences with those of 34 white and minority executives and nonexecutives (managers). Executives were defined as corporate officers or direct reports to corporate officers with responsibility for general management or a core business function, such as division president or vice president/general manager or leadership of a corporate function such as finance (Thomas and Gabarro 1999, 7). The in-depth interviews focused on family background, progression of jobs, developmental experiences, and the effects of race on careers. In addition, the researchers interviewed three people nominated by each participant to share their impressions of that executive. This study is significant because of its depth and insights into minority executive career trajectory experiences in corporate America. I mention it here because this work had a profound influence on me as a researcher and on the design of this study.

Another CEO study examined white women, African Americans, Hispanics/Latinos, and Asian Americans working in Fortune 500 companies (Zweigenhaft and Domhoff 2014). The researchers looked at variables such as whether participants had been promoted internally or recruited externally, education, class background, and skin color. Key findings indicated that most of the participants had strong educational backgrounds, came from the upper middle class or upper third of the social strata, and had been promoted from inside their companies. In addition, the researchers mentioned that the African Americans and Hispanics/Latinos in the study had lighter skin color. In sum, they concluded that a combination of these factors led to their career progression to CEO.

In the healthcare field, studies have examined barriers to career advancement for racially and ethnically diverse professionals. One study conducted focus groups with diverse healthcare managers and asked them six questions related to racial and ethnic disparities in their career advancement (Dreachslin, Jimpson, and Sprainer 2001). Nineteen themes were identified, including "institutionalized racism limits opportunities; lack of mentors limit achievements; African Americans are concentrated in public sector and inner city hospitals with lower pay; people of color are burdened with negative stereotypes; and whites see black achievement as a threat" (Dreachslin, Jimpson, and Sprainer 2001, 403). Another theme indicated that top executives need to make a commitment to diversity leadership. Again, the study emphasized the critical role of C-suite leadership.

In a related study, researchers not only focused on career advancement factors affecting racially and ethnically diverse professionals but also included women (Dreachslin and Curtis 2004). This study examined root causes of career disparities among minority individuals, women, and non-Hispanic white men, especially at the executive level. A comprehensive literature review and interviews with key informants in the field yielded two theoretical frameworks found in the literature: social factors and human capital factors.

Social factors were organized into three categories: social attitudes, socioeconomic differences, and sociopolitical background. Social attitudes were aligned with the previous study, indicating that prejudice, stereotypes, and discrimination affected career advancement. Socioeconomic differences included factors such as education and income. Sociopolitical background included historical racial and ethnic differences in treatment and current environment. The authors (Dreachslin and Curtis 2004) identified these social factors as the root cause of differences in career outcomes for racial and ethnic minorities. They identified human capital factors such as education, experience, technical competencies, and interpersonal competencies. They posited that social factors and human capital factors are synergistic and have a direct impact on health service organizations that, in turn, affect career outcomes.

Similar barriers to advancement were found in a study that focused on the underrepresentation of black American women in healthcare administration (Brown 2015). This study interviewed seven black women in leadership positions who had the potential for promotion to the executive level. Interview results indicated that key barriers to advancement were related to racial issues such as bias and inequities, succession planning exclusion, undervaluing of qualifications, and stereotyping. Another study indicated that underrepresentation in the workplace, whether among women or people of color, often means dealing with the threat of being stereotyped (Block et al. 2011). The threat of negative racial/ethnic and gender stereotypes may affect the performance of those in these social identity groups. Other researchers posited that the "white standard" is the leadership prototype in the United States and influences the performance ratings of racial and ethnic minorities, which may also hinder their career advancement (Rosette, Leonardelli, and Phillips 2008, 759).

ACHE's "Racial/Ethnic Comparison of Career Attainments in Healthcare Management" study asked survey respondents whether they were evaluated according to standards that they believed to be inappropriate (ACHE 2015b, 67). Compared with 6 percent of white respondents, 30 percent of black respondents, 18 percent of Hispanic/Latino respondents, and 16 percent of Asian American respondents believed that inappropriate standards were used in their evaluations. Only 3 percent of white respondents believed that they had not been promoted because of their race/ethnicity, but 39 percent of black, 26 percent of Asian American, and 16 percent of Hispanic/Latino respondents thought this was a factor in their career progression (ACHE 2015b, 67).

These studies shed light on the barriers that racial and ethnic minorities may encounter on the executive path. It is also important to understand the success factors that help them reach CEO and other C-suite positions in healthcare.

CAREER SUCCESS FACTORS

Limited research has been conducted on the success factors that help advance racially and ethnically diverse professionals to the CEO and other C-suite positions in hospitals and health systems. An early survey study of executives who aspired to the CEO position from 54 hospitals in a Western state did not include the race or ethnicity of respondents (Parsons et al. 1997).

ACHE's "Career Attainments in Healthcare Management" study also provides insights into success factors that may influence different career outcomes (ACHE 2015b). Education was a key factor in the participants' career advancement. The majority of survey participants held graduate degrees in health administration or business administration. Participation in fellowships, internships, or residency programs was another important factor related to education and gaining professional experience: approximately 20 percent of the participants who had completed healthcare management residencies and three-quarters who had completed fellowships were hired by the host organization (ACHE 2015b, 9). A high percentage of participants started as department heads. Also, the study found that mentors had a significant impact on early career experiences, with approximately three-fourths of the respondents indicating that they had a mentor. As they gained experience, most respondents changed organizations. Most also participated in professional organizations.

Other studies have focused on how women attained the CEO position in healthcare. In one qualitative study, 35 female healthcare executives were interviewed about their career trajectories (Roemer 2002). Twenty percent of the women were members of a racial/ethnic minority. The majority of study participants were CEOs, but not only in hospitals and health systems. Organizations also included community health centers, home healthcare agencies, health maintenance organizations, and other types of healthcare organizations. In addition, chief operating officers (COOs) were included; two of the participants had previously held CEO positions, and another was in consideration for a CEO position.

Results showed that while 54 percent of the women had mentors, only a small number believed that having or not having mentors played a consequential role in their careers (i.e., believed they were in their position because of the mentor). Another reason for success was the women's capacity to learn, which included obtaining graduate education in management. Hard work and risk taking were other factors. Some participants also cited serendipity—being in the right place at the right time—as a factor in their career progression.

More recently, Donald Sexton, Christy Lemak, and Joyce Wainio (2014) studied the career trajectories of 20 successful women hospital CEOs. This study included racially and ethnically diverse women, with three African Americans and two Hispanics/Latinas. The sample included two COOs who had previously been CEOs. The researchers examined "career inflection points"—that is, points of significant change, either positive or negative, on the career path (Sexton, Lemak, and Wainio 2014, 370). The findings identified 25 inflection points categorized by six key themes: education and training, experience, career management, family, networking, and mentorship and sponsorship. There were differences in career turning points among the women who worked in healthcare management and in clinical or administrative support positions. Graduate education and COO experience were consistently cited by all the study participants.

These studies provide some understanding of the career experiences that influence movement on the career path to CEO and other C-suite positions. Opportunities remain to learn more from female and male racial and ethnic minorities about their experiences on the executive path and the leadership competencies that accelerated their progression. Effective leadership is essential for professionals who seek C-suite positions.

Effective leadership has been defined in many ways, and the definitions have been debated in the academic and practitioner literature. For the purposes of this research, Dr. John Kotter's definition indicates that leadership moves people to a better place without creating harm to others through constructive or adaptive change (Kotter 1990, 5). He suggests that leadership occurs through establishing direction, aligning people, and motivating and inspiring. This description of leadership is aligned with the competency domain in the Healthcare Leadership Alliance's competency model (Garman, Butler, and Brinkmeyer 2006; Stefl 2008). In this model, leadership is defined as "the ability to inspire individual and organizational excellence, to create and attain a shared vision, and to successfully manage change to attain the organization's strategic ends and successful performance" (Stefl 2008, 364). Leadership intersects with four other competency domains: communication and relationship management, professionalism, knowledge of healthcare environment, and business knowledge and skills (Stefl 2008, 365).

The "ACHE Healthcare Executive 2019 Competencies Assessment Tool" further defines leadership as encompassing leadership skills and behavior, organizational climate and culture, communicating vision, and managing change (HLA and ACHE 2019). The literature does not specifically identify leadership competencies that facilitate career advancement to the CEO position for racially and ethnically diverse professionals.

STUDY PURPOSE

The purpose of this study was to deepen understanding of the career trajectory experiences and leadership competencies that facilitated the advancement of racially and ethnically diverse professionals to the CEO position. There were two key objectives:

- To describe the significant career trajectory experiences on the executive path that led to the CEO position.
- To describe the leadership competencies that facilitated advancement on the executive path to CEO.

Understanding the executive path journey to CEO can yield valuable insights that can be translated into executive development and organizational change strategies that will help minorities achieve C-suite and other executive positions in healthcare.

METHODOLOGY

Study Sample

The study sample comprised 12 racial/ethnic minority hospital and health system CEOs. Racial/ethnic minorities encompass individuals who are not categorized as "non-Hispanic white alone" according to the US Census Bureau (Colby and Ortman 2015; US Census Bureau 2017). Projections for the composition of the US population indicate that the non-Hispanic white population is still the majority group at the time of this writing. However, the categorizations of "majority" and "minority" are projected to change by 2044, when the US population will be made up of a plurality of racial and ethnic groups (Colby and Ortman 2015). Currently, the minority population includes black or African Americans, American Indians and Alaska Natives, Asians, Native Hawaiian and Other Pacific Islanders, and people of Hispanic/Latino origin. Hispanic is designated as an ethnicity by the Census Bureau, and people of this origin may be of any race (US Census Bureau 2017).

In addition, the term "minority" is used to signify that this segment of the population remains a minority in the C-suites of hospitals and health systems (ACHE 2015b; Institute for Diversity and Health Equity 2015). The 12 executives interviewed for this research include four African Americans, four Hispanics/Latinos, and four Asian Americans, with two men and two women in each group.

This qualitative phenomenological research study was designed to achieve an in-depth understanding of the career trajectory experiences of these executives, including the leadership competencies that facilitated the progression of racially and ethnically diverse CEOs on the executive path. Qualitative methods can provide rich information that describes and illuminates the experiences of individuals or groups, contributing knowledge to the health services field for practical application (Sofaer 1999). In qualitative inquiry, there are no set parameters for sample size (Patton 1990). The size of the sample depends on several criteria: what the researcher wants to know, the purpose of the inquiry, usefulness, credibility, and what can be accomplished with time and resources available (Patton 1990, 184). It was determined that a sample of 12 individuals with equal representation of racial and ethnic minority groups and gender would meet these criteria.

Only active racial and ethnic hospital and health system CEOs or the equivalent were eligible to participate—the top C-suite executive of the entity. All CEOs were active at the time they agreed to participate in the study. However, in one case, a CEO took another executive position outside the hospital setting by the time of the interview, but this individual had been an active CEO at that hospital for seven years.

A hospital may be an individual entity or part of a health system that is composed of more than one hospital. In some health systems, the top executive of a hospital entity may not have the CEO title. Titles in these situations were president or administrator. Also, the hospital top executive within a health system often has additional responsibilities within the system beyond the individual entity.

Study participants were identified through a purposeful sampling process. Specifically, snowball or chain sampling was used to identify information-rich cases (Patton 1990). This approach involved asking well-connected professionals in the healthcare field whom they knew that could provide meaningful information and be open to participating in this type of study. In addition, several sources were reviewed, such as *Modern Healthcare*'s "Top 25 Minority Executives in Healthcare," *Healthcare Executive*, the *Journal of Healthcare Management*, the Furst Group's "C-Suite Conversations," *Becker's Hospital Review*, and *Hospitals & Health Networks* magazine.

Each prospective participant's background was examined. In addition to racial/ethnic group and gender, a combination of factors influenced selection, including the type of hospital or health system: for-profit or not-for-profit. The majority of participants came from different types of not-for-profit hospitals and health systems. One individual was the CEO of a for-profit health system. The other study participants worked for not-for-profit health systems but had previous experiences in for-profit systems. The intent of the selection process was to include a variety of backgrounds, if possible.

After the list of potential participants was developed, the recruitment procedure was designed. A one-page study description was prepared before contacting the CEOs. Prior to calling or emailing potential participants, approval was sought from the University of Maryland's Institutional Review Board (IRB). The study received expedited review status and was determined to be a minimal-risk project, but based on the risks, the project had to be reviewed by the IRB committee on an annual basis. In all, 19 CEOs were contacted.

In most cases, the CEO's executive assistant was contacted by telephone and given a brief explanation of the research study. The assistant was then asked to share the one-page study description with the CEO. If the CEO was interested, in most cases, a 15-minute telephone conversation was scheduled to describe the study in more depth and answer any questions. Also, the IRB Consent Form was explained. In three cases, the CEOs were contacted directly by email or telephone. After a commitment was obtained, the researcher worked with the CEO's executive assistant to schedule the interview and to obtain the CEO's signature on the IRB Consent Form. Two CEOs who initially committed to participate dropped out of the study because of scheduling conflicts. They were replaced, resulting in a final sample size of 12 participants.

The background characteristics of the participants are detailed in appendix B. Participants were equally represented across racial/ethnic minority groups and genders—four African Americans (two women, two men), four Hispanics/Latinos (two women, two men), and four Asian Americans (two women, two men). One participant had come to the United States without parents as an exchange student and remained to obtain a college education. Another emigrated to this country with parents as a child. Their ages ranged from 44 to 64 years.

All had graduate degrees, with the majority attaining master of health or healthcare administration (MHA) degrees. A nurse also had a master of nursing degree. Three participants had master of business administration (MBA) degrees; one was a dual degree with an MHA, and in another case, a physician had gone back to school to obtain an MBA. See appendix B for additional information about specific degrees.

The functional backgrounds included five participants from clinical areas—one nurse, one physician, two physical therapy professionals, and one medical technologist—and five with general healthcare administration backgrounds. In addition, one participant had an accounting and industrial engineering background, and one was an attorney.

The CEOs came from different geographic locations in the United States: Four were located on the East Coast, one in the Midwest, four in the Southwest, and three on the West Coast. The locations are not aligned with specific participants in an effort to protect their identities.

Data Collection

In-depth, face-to-face semistructured interviews were conducted with the CEOs in their offices between September 2016 and June 2017. A phenomenological research method was used to understand the lived experiences on the executive path for the purpose of gaining insights into the leadership competencies and significant career trajectory experiences that led to the CEO position (Moustakas 1994; van Manen 2007). Interviews sought to understand the participants' point of view and uncover the meaning of their lived experiences (Kvale 1996).

The interview protocol consisted of two 90-minute meetings that were designed to gather data in a manner that allowed the CEOs to describe their experiences. These experiences included the progression of jobs, leadership development programs, developmental relationships, career setbacks and mistakes, racial/ethnic-related experiences that affected their careers, leadership competencies, and lessons learned (Thomas and Gabarro 1999). This protocol involved asking open-ended questions that were prepared in advance and engaging in dialogue with the participants during the interviews—but, most importantly, listening and learning (Moustakas 1994).

Preparation for the interviews was important for both the interviewer and the participants. "Epoche" was a valuable process for the interviewer (Moustakas 1994, 85). Epoche involves making every effort to set aside prejudgments, preconceived ideas, and biases to be as open-minded as possible during the interviews. In this case, the researcher was mindful of the risk of prejudging results and consciously reflected on preconceived ideas or theories about the executive path, documenting them so that they would not be forgotten during the research process. The phenomenological method realistically does not seek to disconnect from all ideas previously ascertained but rather to set them aside in a manner that enables new knowledge and perspectives to be learned (Moustakas 1994, 85). This method suggests entering the interviewing process with a mindset of wonder, being motivated by fascination with learning (van Manen 2007).

Participant preparation for the two in-depth interviews involved asking each CEO to share information such as a résumé or curriculum vitae that outlined their background and career progression. In addition, they were sent an Interview Preparation Guide and asked to reflect on their career progression and significant experiences. It was evident that most of the participants had prepared for the interviews. This helped the interviewer obtain rich descriptions of the participants' experiences on the executive path.

In the first part of the interview, the initial meeting focused on gathering background information and inquiry about career progression using the individual's résumé or curriculum vitae as a guide. As the participants described each position they had held, they were asked about significant accomplishments, developmental relationships, leadership development, leadership competencies that facilitated advancement, career setbacks and mistakes, other significant experiences, career/life balance, and lessons learned that impacted their career journey during that time.

The second part of the interview was conducted the next day for the CEOs who were not within driving distance. For those who were within driving distance, the interview was scheduled for the following week. The second meeting typically began with participants reflecting on the first interview and providing any additional information about their career progression. Next, the questions examined whether the executives' race/ethnicity had affected their advancement and leadership approach. Most of the interviews concluded with open-ended inquiry about additional reflections the participants wanted to share about experiences and thoughts on the research. Interviews were recorded using an Olympus digital voice recorder. Field notes were also taken during each interview.

Although gender was not the focus of this study, several of the women interviewed talked about the impact of gender on their careers. It is difficult to separate racial/ethnic identity from gender identity because of the intersectionality of race and gender (Chin, Desormeaux, and Sawyer 2016; Crenshaw 1989). Experiences of being a racially/ethnically diverse professional and a woman are not mutually exclusive but rather are intertwined and interact (Crenshaw 1989).

In keeping with IRB ethics standards, the interview data remain confidential. The actual names and locations of the study participants have been disguised. Confidentiality of the data collected was managed by refraining from using the real names and work locations of the study participants in verbal communications and publications about the research.

DATA ANALYSIS

All interview tapes were transcribed verbatim. It was important to be mindful of prejudgments, biases, and preconceived ideas to ensure that the participants' actual words were transcribed, without being affected by the researcher's interpretation (Moustakas 1994). The researcher listened to the tapes several times and compared the tapes with the written text to check for accuracy.

Listening to the tapes enabled the researcher to obtain a general understanding of the data; notes were taken as rudimentary themes emerged. It was imperative to keep in mind the purpose of the research and the specific topics being investigated. The bracketed focus helped with phenomenological reduction, in which the text is described just as it was to discern meanings and essences (Moustakas 1994; van Manen 2007). The process of repeatedly and consciously reflecting and concentrating on new perspectives and ideas that surfaced yielded moments of insightful meaning. Initially, everything had equal value, so that the whole understanding of the executive path experience, including leadership competencies, could be identified. Gradually and decisively, insightful meanings were organized into the clusters of invariant themes.

A related qualitative method is content analysis, which involves coding and categorizing primary patterns in the interview texts (Patton 1990). It was important to compare the invariant themes derived through the phenomenological method with the results of the patterns identified through the coding process to enhance rigor. Coding involved reading and rereading all of the interview transcripts. Topics were identified using different colored highlighters to label the text and writing notes in the margins of the transcripts. File cards were used to develop a system to organize the key topics. These key topics were compared with the invariant themes identified earlier, verifying the reliability of the results. The themes were reconciled, bringing out the essence of the participants' experiences on the executive path.

Some people might question this approach from a strictly phenomenological perspective. Further, some might question why qualitative data analysis software (QDAS) was not used to identify themes. Some phenomenological scholars, such as Max van Manen (2014, 319), believe that "codifications, conceptual abstractions, or empirical generalizations can never adequately produce phenomenological understandings and insights." Others believe these methods of analysis do not diminish the efficacy of phenomenological research (Goble et al. 2012; Sohn 2017). Specifically, for this research, QDAS was not used because the sample size of 12 was small enough to engage in theme analysis without being overwhelmed by the data. With regard to coding, this researcher agrees that there is value in looking at the data more than one way by using mixed strategies with the intent of strengthening the study (Patton 1990).

An additional step in reflective analysis consists of going deeper to discover structures of meanings through "imaginative variation" (Moustakas, 1994, 97–99). This step involves recognizing variations in meanings and themes, such as those between women and men. Also, it involves looking for examples that illustrate, explain, or support the invariant themes, such as using participant quotations that support the themes. In addition, working to uncover the underlying reasons for the feelings and thoughts that were expressed deepened understanding of the "heart of things"—the very essence of meaning (van Manen 2007). To facilitate this process, the researcher thought about the essences of the executive path that made a difference in the career trajectories of the participants and the leadership competencies that helped these minority CEOs advance.

The final phase of analysis involved the synthesis of essences and meanings—although reflection and learning are ongoing. Moustakas (1994, 100) notes that "the essences of any experience are never totally exhausted." It was important to integrate the descriptions of the executive path experiences and leadership competencies to create a composite understanding of the whole experience.

ADDRESSING THE CHALLENGES OF QUALITATIVE RESEARCH

One of the key challenges of qualitative research is determining whether the researcher's attitude, prejudices, and assumptions affected the conduct of the research inquiry and analysis. As mentioned earlier, from the phenomenological method perspective, the researcher was mindful of attitudes, biases, and preconceived ideas about the research topic and made efforts to consciously set aside prejudices and preconceptions (Moustakas 1994; van Manen 2014). While it is not possible to set aside all preconceived thinking and background, the researcher consciously and mindfully identified what could interfere with being open to learning new knowledge.

Reflexivity suggests that "the researcher's background and position will affect what they choose to investigate, the angle of the investigation, the methods judged most adequate for this purpose, the findings considered most appropriate, and the framing and communication of conclusions" (Malterud 2001, 483–84). For this reason, it was important for this researcher to acknowledge that a study of hospital CEOs' transformational leadership had been conducted previously. How learning obtained from that study affected the current research had to be recognized—that is, hospital CEOs' balance of transformational and transactional leadership approaches affected aspects of hospital effectiveness. It was critical to recognize how this knowledge could affect the interviewing process and data analysis. In addition, as a leadership and organization development consultant and lecturer on transformational leadership in healthcare, preconceptions based on theory and practical experiences may have framed the researcher's understanding of leadership. Further, the researcher has previous experience working in a health system with executives including CEOs and managers at all levels that could affect objectivity.

Malterud (2001, 484) indicates that "subjectivity arises when the effect of the researcher is ignored." It was essential to consider how these frames of reference and background created preconceptions that might impact the current study. Of note is a perspective that biases are not the same as preconceptions as long as the researcher understands and acknowledges them (Malterud 2001). This perspective goes further to posit that "personal issues can be valuable sources for relevant and specific research" (Malterud 2001, 484). This researcher believed that her background and experiences were valuable and useful for designing the study, gaining access to the CEOs, interviewing the participants, and analyzing the data. However, efforts were made during every phase of the research process to be mindful of the researcher's potential biases and how they might affect constructing what was being learned.

An additional step taken to address reflexivity was to engage an outsider to discuss the research process. This person was a former professor who taught qualitative research and has conducted numerous qualitative studies outside the healthcare field. He provided impartial viewpoints and guidance on the study. During three meetings, the research, qualitative analysis methods, and a draft research report were discussed. Feedback was received in each of these areas.

LIMITATIONS

All research studies have limitations. This study's results are not generalizable from the standpoint of drawing conclusions from the sample of 12 racially and ethnically diverse hospital and health system CEOs and generalizing them to the population of all minority healthcare CEOs and the population of hospital and health system CEOs. Phenomenological study findings do not result in empirical generalizations (van Manen 2014). It is possible, however, to discern generalized insights about the CEOs' career trajectory experiences and leadership competencies that accelerated advancement on the executive path.

The scope of this study was limited by financial resources and the time it would have taken to include other racial groups in the research. For example, racial groups such as American Indians or

Alaska Natives and Native Hawaiians or other Pacific Islanders were not included in the study sample. In addition, executives belonging to two or more racial groups were not studied.

The research did not incorporate white women and men. A comparison of the career trajectory experiences of white women and men with racially and ethnically diverse professionals on the executive path would provide additional insights into similarities and differences in career experiences.

These limitations provide opportunities for future research.

REFERENCES

American College of Healthcare Executives (ACHE). 2015a. "Increasing and Sustaining Racial/Ethnic Diversity in Health-care Management." Policy statement. Revised November. www.ache.org/about-ache/our-story/our-commitments/policy-statements/increasing-and-sustaining-racial-diversity-in-healthcare-management.

———. 2015b. "A Racial/Ethnic Comparison of Career Attainments in Healthcare Management." Published January. www.ache.org/-/media/ache/learning-center/research/2014raceethnicityreport.pdf.

Block, C. J., S. M. Koch, B. E. Liberman, T. J. Merriweather, and L. Roberson. 2011. "Contending with Stereotype Threat at Work: A Model of Long-Term Responses." *Counseling Psychologist* 39 (4): 570–600.

Brown, A. L. 2015. "Factors Relating to Underrepresentation of Black American Women in Health Care Administration." PhD diss., Walden University.

Carmeli, A., J. Schaubroeck, and A. Tishler. 2011. "How CEO Empowering Leadership Shapes Top Management Team Processes: Implications for Firm Performance." *Leadership Quarterly* 22 (2): 399–411.

Chin, J. L., L. Desormeaux, and K. Sawyer. 2016. "Making Way for Paradigms of Diversity Leadership." *Consulting Psychology Journal: Practice and Research* 68 (1): 49–71.

Colby, S. L., and J. M. Ortman. 2015. "Projections of the Size and Composition of the US Population: 2014 to 2060." US Census Bureau current population report. Published March. www.census.gov/content/dam/Census/library/publications/2015/demo/p25-1143.pdf.

Crenshaw, K. 1989. "Demarginalizing the Intersection of Race and Sex: A Black Feminist Critique of Antidiscrimination Doctrine, Feminist Theory, and Antiracist Politics." *University of Chicago Legal Forum* 140: 139–67.

Dansky, K. H., R. Weech-Maldonado, G. DeSouza, and J. L. Dreachslin. 2003. "Organizational Strategy and Diversity Management: Diversity-Sensitive Orientation as a Moderating Influence." *Health Care Management Review* 28 (3): 243–53.

Dixon, D. L. 1997. "The Relationship Between Chief Executive Leadership (Transactional and Transformational) and Hospital Effectiveness." EdD diss., George Washington University.

Dolan, T. C. 2013. "Increasing Diversity in Governance and Management." *Journal of Healthcare Management* 58 (2): 84–86.

Dotson, E., and A. Nuru-Jeter. 2012. "Setting the Stage for a Business Case for Leadership Diversity in Healthcare: History, Research, and Leverage." *Journal of Healthcare Management* 57 (1): 35–43.

Dreachslin, J. L. 2007a. "Diversity Management and Cultural Competence: Research, Practice, and the Business Case." *Journal of Healthcare Management* 52 (2): 79–86.

———. 2007b. "The Role of Leadership in Creating a Diversity-Sensitive Organization." *Journal of Healthcare Management* 52 (3): 151–55.

————. 1999. "Diversity Leadership and Organizational Transformation: Performance Indicators for Health Services Organizations." *Journal of Healthcare Management* 44 (6): 427–39.

Dreachslin, J. L., and E. F. Curtis. 2004. "Study of Factors Affecting the Career Advancement of Women and Racially/Ethnically Diverse Individuals in Healthcare Management." *Journal of Health Administration Education* 21 (4): 441–84.

Dreachslin, J. L., and F. Hobby. 2008. "Racial and Ethnic Disparities: Why Diversity Leaders Matter." *Journal of Healthcare Management* 53 (1): 8–13.

Dreachslin, J. L., G. E. Jimpson, and E. Sprainer. 2001. "Race, Ethnicity and Careers in Healthcare Management." *Journal of Healthcare Management* 46 (6): 397–409.

Dreachslin, J. L., R. Weech-Maldonado, and K. H. Dansky. 2004. "Racial and Ethnic Diversity and Organizational Behavior: A Focused Research Agenda for Health Services Management." *Social Science & Medicine* 59 (5): 961–71.

Dreachslin, J. L., R. Weech-Maldonado, J. Gail, J. P. Epane, and J. A. Wainio. 2017. "Blueprint for Sustainable Change in Diversity Management and Cultural Competence: Lessons from the National Center for Healthcare Leadership Demonstration Project." *Journal of Healthcare Management* 62 (3): 171–82.

Eagly, A. H., and J. L. Chin. 2010. "Diversity and Leadership in a Changing World." *American Psychologist* 65 (3): 216–24.

Finkelstein, S., and D. C. Hambrick. 1996. *Strategic Leadership: Top Executives and Their Effects on Organizations*. Minneapolis–St. Paul, MN: West Publishing Company.

Flores, K., and G. Combs. 2013. "Minority Representation in Healthcare: Increasing the Number of Professionals Through Focused Recruitment." *Hospital Topics* 91 (2): 25–36.

Garman, A. N., P. Butler, and L. Brinkmeyer. 2006. "Leadership." *Journal of Healthcare Management* 51 (6): 360–64.

Goble, E., W. Austin, D. Larsen, L. Kreitzer, and S. Brintnell. 2012. "Habits of Mind and the Split-Mind Effect: When Computer-Assisted Qualitative Data Analysis Software Is Used in Phenomenological Research." *Forum: Qualitative Social Research.* Accessed June 5, 2019. www.qualitative-research.net/index.php/fqs/article/view/1709/3340.

Hambrick, D. C. 2007. "Upper Echelons Theory: An Update." *Academy of Management Review* 32 (2): 334–43.

Hambrick, D. C., and P. A. Mason. 1984. "Upper Echelons: The Organization as a Reflection of Its Top Managers." *Academy of Management Review* 9 (2): 193–206.

Hambrick, D. C., and T. J. Quigley. 2014. "Toward More Accurate Contextualization of the CEO Effect on Firm Performance." *Strategic Management Journal* 35 (4): 473–91.

Healthcare Leadership Alliance (HLA) and American College of Healthcare Executives (ACHE). 2019. "ACHE Healthcare Executive 2019 Competencies Assessment Tool." Accessed May 29. www.ache.org/-/media/ache/career-resource-center/competencies_booklet.pdf.

Institute for Diversity and Health Equity. 2015. "Diversity and Disparities: A Benchmark Study of US Hospitals in 2015." Accessed June 5, 2019. www.diversityconnection.org/diversityconnection/leadership-conferences/Benchmarking-Survey.jsp.

Kotter, J. P. 1990. *A Force for Change: How Leadership Differs from Management.* New York: Free Press.

Kvale, S. 1996. *Inter View: An Introduction to Qualitative Research Interviewing.* Thousand Oaks, CA: Sage Publications.

Malterud, K. 2001. "Qualitative Research: Standards, Challenges, and Guidelines." *The Lancet* 358 (9280): 483–88.

Moustakas, C. 1994. *Phenomenological Research Methods*. Thousand Oaks, CA: Sage Publications.

Parsons, R. J., G. Gustafson, B. P. Murray, R. B. Dwore, P. Smith, and L. H. Vorderer. 1997. "Hospital Administrators' Career Paths: Which Way to the Top." *Health Care Management Review* 22 (4): 82–92.

Patton, M. Q. 1990. *Qualitative Evaluation and Research Methods*, 2nd ed. Newbury Park, CA: Sage Publications.

Roemer, L. 2002. "Women CEOs in Health Care: Did They Have Mentors?" *Health Care Management Review* 27 (4): 57–67.

Rosenbach, W. E., M. Sashkin, and F. Harburg. 1996. *The Leadership Profile: On Becoming a Better Leader*. Seabrook, MD: Ducochon Press.

Rosette, A. S., G. J. Leonardelli, and K. W. Phillips. 2008. "The White Standard: Racial Bias in Leader Categorization." *Journal of Applied Psychology* 93 (4): 758–77.

Schein, E. H. 2010. *Organizational Culture and Leadership*. San Francisco: John Wiley & Sons.

Sexton, D. W., C. H. Lemak, and J. A. Wainio. 2014. "Career Inflection Points of Women Who Successfully Achieved the Hospital CEO Position." *Journal of Healthcare Management* 59 (5): 367–84.

Sofaer, S. 1999. "Qualitative Methods: What Are They and Why Use Them?" *Health Services Research* 34 (5): 1101–18.

Sohn, B. K. 2017. "Phenomenology and Qualitative Data Analysis Software (QDAS): A Careful Reconciliation." *Forum: Qualitative*

Social Research. Accessed June 5, 2019. www.qualitative-research.net/index.php/fqs/article/view/2688.

Stefl, M. E. 2008. "Common Competencies for All Healthcare Managers: The Healthcare Leadership Alliance Model." *Journal of Healthcare Management* 53 (6): 360–72.

Thomas, D. A., and J. J. Gabarro. 1999. *Breaking Through: The Making of Minority Executives in Corporate America*. Boston: Harvard Business School Press.

US Bureau of Labor Statistics. 2017. "Employment Projections: 2016–26 Summary." Published October 24. www.bls.gov/news.release/ecopro.nr0.htm.

US Census Bureau. 2017. "Race & Ethnicity." Published January. www.census.gov/mso/www/training/pdf/race-ethnicity-one pager.pdf.

van Manen, M. 2014. *Phenomenology of Practice: Meaning-Giving Methods in Phenomenological Research and Writing*. New York: Taylor & Francis.

———. 2007. "Phenomenology of Practice." *Phenomenology & Practice* 1 (1): 11–30.

Witt/Kieffer. 2011. "Building the Business Case. Healthcare Diversity Leadership: A National Survey Report." Accessed June 5, 2019. www.wittkieffer.com/file/thought-leadership/practice/Diversity%20as%20a%20business%20builder_2011.pdf.

Zweigenhaft, R. L., and G. W. Domhoff. 2014. *The New CEOs*. Lanham, MD: Rowman & Littlefield.

Study Participant Background Characteristics

Race/ethnicity and gender (*n*)	Functional background (*n*)
African American (4)	Clinical (5)
Women (2)	Nurse (1)
Men (2)	Physician (1)
Hispanic/Latino (4)	Physical therapist (2)
Women (2)	Medical technologist (1)
Men (2)	Legal—attorney (1)
Asian American (4)	Accounting and industrial
Women (2)	engineering (1)
Men (2)	Healthcare administration (5)
Age (*n*)	**Organization type (*n*)**
44–48 years (3)	Not-for-profit (11)
52–56 years (5)	Hospital within health
61–64 years (4)	system (3)
	Academic medical center (3)
	Comprehensive health
	system (2)
	Public hospital system (3)
	For-profit market/system (1)

(continued)

(continued from previous page)

Education (*n*)	Geographic location (*n*)
MHA (4)	East Coast (4)
MPA and certificate in health services administration (1)	Midwest (1)
	Southwest (4)
MPH (1)	West Coast (3)
MHA/MBA (1)	
MD and MBA (1)	
Master of accountancy and MBA (1)	
MSN and MHA (1)	
MS (1)	
JD (1)	

Index

Note: Italicized page locators refer to exhibits.

136–37, *145*; developing and maintaining relationships, 133–34, *145*; effective communication, 134–36, *145*; emotional intelligence, 131–32, *145*; engagement of people at all levels, 137–38, *145*; financial and business acumen, 143–44, *145*; leading and managing organizational change, 140–41, *145*; leading with vision, 139, *145*; learning mindfully, 132–33, *145*; organizing framework for, *145*; overview of, 130–31; political acumen, 142–43, *145*; team development, 138–39, *145*

Leadership development: intentional nature of, 89; "stretch" assignments and, 35

Leadership opportunities: sponsors and, 68

Lean Six Sigma, 140

Learning: family and emphasis on, 1–2; "leaderly," 133; mindful, 77, 117, 132–33, 152, *153*, 156–57; openness to, 35, 36–37, *40*, 47, 133. *See also* Education

Learning as a Way of Being (Vaill), 133

Learning mindset: executives' comments on, 101–2, 103

Learning opportunities: challenges, mistakes, and setbacks as, 121, 123

Lemak, Christy, 172

Limiting assignments, 110–11

LinkedIn, 96

Listening, 36, 135

Loyalty: early lessons about, 2

Malik, Rubina, 61

Malterud, K., 182

Management: leadership vs., 126–27, 145–46; relationship, importance of, 133–34

Master of business administration (MBA) degree, 4, 177, 192

Master of health/healthcare administration (MHA) degree, 4, 177, 192

Master of public health (MPH) degree, 4

Master of science in nursing (MSN) degree, 4, 177, 192

Meaningful relationships, 45–46

Meditation, 122

Mentoring: cross-race, 54–55

Mentors, 12, 29, 51–55, 69, 82; alternative perspectives on, 53–54; bosses as, 46; career advancement and role of, 51–52; career success for women and, 172; collaboration skills and, 136; communication skills and, 93; descriptions of, 51–52; mistakes made and seeking support from, 118, 119; as personal advisers, 159; professional demeanor tips and, 92; race/ethnicity in relationships with, 54–55; reasons for, 52; seeking, 152, *153*, 156; working with, 52–53. *See also* Sponsors

Mentorship: attainment of sponsorship vs., 62

Mettle: emotional intelligence and, 132

Microaggressions: definition of, 17; managing, 23

Mindful learning, 77, 117, 132–33, 152, *153*, 156–57

Mindset: definition of, 101

Minorities. *See* Race and ethnicity

Minority CEOs: career advancement and, 167–70

Minority men: white men vs., career attainments in healthcare management and, 165

Mission: "best you" and, 164; executive path and, 89; redefined C-suite and, 163; vision aligned with, 139; wisdom and, 159

Mistakes and career setbacks, rebounding from, 84, 116–22; admitting to mistakes, 30; "jumping into the deep end without a life preserver," 117–18; key themes for, 121–22; political mistakes, 118–19; taking a wrong turn, 116–17; types of mistakes and setbacks, learning from, 119–21

Modern Healthcare: "Top 25 Minority Executives in Healthcare," 175

Moustakas, C., 181

National Association of Health Services Executives (NAHSE), 96, 97

Native Hawaiians, 174, 183

Negative communication approach, 109

Private sector corporations: emerging, changing C-suite and, 162

Professional associations, 95–96, 97

Professional demeanor: cultivating, 92, 102

Promotions: failures in, 108–9; performance excellence and, 100; reasons for changing positions and, 84; sponsors and, 55

Protégés: roles and responsibilities of, 71–72

Purpose, 82; clarity of, 81; focus on, 23

Qualitative data analysis software (QDAS), 181

Qualitative inquiry: sample size and, 175

Qualitative phenomenological research study: addressing challenges of qualitative research, 182–83; data analysis, 180–81; data collection, 177–79; limitations of, 183–84; methodology, 174–79; participant background characteristics, 176–77, 191–92; purpose of, 173–74; research overview, 165–73; study sample, 174–77; two key objectives in, xiv, 173

Race and ethnicity: addressing diversity of leaders in terms of, 128–29; barriers to career advancement and, themes in studies on, 169; career success factors and, 171–73; comments on leadership approach, 20–22; conscious/unconscious biases about, 65, 66–67, 71; intersectionality of gender and race, 10, 179; in mentoring relationships, 54–55; networking insights and, 97–98, 102; question of over-mentored and under-sponsored, 62; reflection and action, 25; of research study participants, 174, 176, 191; root causes of career disparities study, 169; self-presentation and, 93; sponsored upward mobility and, 63–64; sponsorship and, 64–65; working with executive recruiters, 87–88. *See also individual racial and ethnic groups*

Race and ethnicity, challenges on executive path: gender more than race, 16–17; no challenges, 17–18; situations that presented challenges, 18–20

Race and ethnicity, reflections on, 9–25; different experiences from those of white counterparts, 14–16; diverse geographic region or organization, 13; executive commentary, 23–24; hard work and performance, 10–11; key lessons, 23; mentors, 12; positive outlook, 13–14; seeking common ground, 11–12

"Racial/Ethnic Comparison of Career Attainments in Healthcare Management" (American College of Healthcare Executives), 165, 170, 171

Racism: institutional, 169; structural, 15

Raju, Ram: on leadership, 146; on potential recognized by sponsor, 73; on turning a crisis into an opportunity, 124

Readiness to make a move: assessing, 85

References: informal networks and, 99

Reflection: on leadership and personal development, 158; navigating executive path journey and, 88, 89; next moves and, 84. *See also* Discernment

Reflective analysis, 180–81

Reflexivity: addressing, 182, 183

Relationship management, 133–34, *145*; bridge building vs., 141–42; engagement and, 137

Relationships: bosses, 46–47; developmental, 46, 50–55; executive coaches, 50–51; executive commentary, 57; key lessons, 56; meaningful, 45–46; mentors, 51–55; peers and colleagues, 47–48; physicians, critical partnerships with, 48–50; power of, 45–58; reflection and action, 58; sponsors, 55; summing up, 55–56

Religious faith: early lessons and impact on, 2

Relocations: career advancement and, 86

Reputation, 99, 109

About the Author

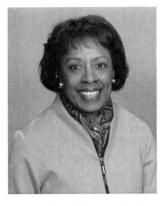

Diane L. Dixon, EdD, is a leadership and organization development educator and consultant. She has more than 30 years of experience in the field of human and organizational learning, focusing on leadership and organization development, managing change and transitions, team development, and training and staff education in organizations of various sizes and complexity. Diane has also worked with nonprofit boards at different stages of strategic planning. She has served on the boards of organizations such as Broadmead Life Plan Retirement Community and Grassroots Crisis Intervention Center.

Before becoming a consultant, Diane was director of human resource development for the former Helix Health System (Union Memorial Hospital and Franklin Square Hospital Center, now part of MedStar Health) and worked in training and development positions for two global corporations, McCormick & Company and Warner-Lambert, Parke-Davis Group.

Diane is a lecturer at the University of Maryland School of Public Health, where she has taught healthcare leadership and communications for the Master of Health Administration Program. Previously, she was an adjunct instructor at Johns Hopkins University, where she taught leadership and organizational behavior in the former Business of Medicine Program and business communication in the Carey Business School. She was faculty for an academic partnership of Johns Hopkins University and America's Health Insurance Plans' (AHIP's) former Minority Management Development Program for six years.

Diane has given numerous leadership presentations focused on transformational leadership and managing organizational change and transitions. She has also presented on board diversity and inclusion for the International Leadership Association. Other presentations include "Effective Leadership in Complex Change and Transitions" for the AHIP Human Resource Leadership Council Meeting and a webinar on the "Impact of Cultural Diversity in the Global Workplace" for AHIP's Information Technology Advisory Group.

For eight years, Diane wrote a monthly leadership column in *Caring for the Ages*, a publication of the American Medical Directors Association. She has contributed chapters on healthcare leadership to three books. In addition, she has written articles for publications such as *Healthcare Forum Journal, Hospitals & Health Networks, Health Progress, Trustee* magazine, the *Journal of Nursing Administration*, and the *Journal of Social Work in Long-Term Care*.

Diane holds a doctorate in education from the Executive Leadership in Human and Organizational Learning Program at George Washington University, where her dissertation research focused on "The Relationship Between Chief Executive Leadership (Transactional and Transformational) and Hospital Effectiveness"; a master of education degree in administration from Loyola University Maryland; and a bachelor of arts in sociology from Howard University.